Vegan Menu for People with Diabetes

Also by Chef Nancy Berkoff, RD

Vegan Microwave Cookbook

Vegan Passover Recipes

Vegan Meals for One or Two

Vegan in Volume

Dedication

This book is dedicated to Dr. Reg Yeske.
He has kept my family healthy and is never too busy
to listen, help, and encourage.

Vegan Menu for People with Diabetes

By Nancy Berkoff, EdD, RD, CCE

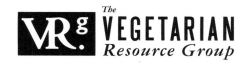

The Vegetarian Resource Group
Baltimore, Maryland

A Note to the Reader

The contents of *Vegan Menu for People with Diabetes* and our other publications, including web information, are not intended to provide personal medical advice. Medical advice should be obtained from a qualified health professional. We often depend on product and ingredient information from company statements. It is impossible to be 100% sure about a statement, information can change, people have different views, and mistakes can be made. Please use your own best judgement about whether a product is suitable for you. To be sure, do further research or confirmation on your own.

© Copyright 2004, The Vegetarian Resource Group
PO Box 1463, Baltimore, MD 21203.

Cover artwork and illustrations by Keryl Cryer

Library of Congress Cataloging-in-Publication Data

Berkoff, Nancy.
  Vegan menu for people with diabetes / by Nancy Berkoff.
      p. cm.
Includes index.
  ISBN 0-931411-28-9 (pbk.)
  1. Diabetes--Diet therapy--recipes. 2. Vegetarian cookery.
  I. Title.
  RC662.B415 2004
  616.4'620654--dc22

                                              2004005629

Printed in the United States of America

10 9 8 7 6 5 4 3 2

Table of Contents

Foreword

APPROXIMATELY 17 MILLION PEOPLE in the United States, or 6.2% of the population, have diabetes; many more are at risk for this disease. Can someone with diabetes follow a vegan diet? Absolutely! A well-planned vegan diet can reduce the risk of heart disease—a disease that those with diabetes are especially prone to develop. A vegan diet that is low in saturated fat and cholesterol and high in fiber and phytochemicals can help to reduce the risk of developing diabetes, particularly when combined with exercise and weight loss (if necessary). These menus make following a vegan diet easy both for people with diabetes and those who are concerned about developing diabetes.

-Reed Mangels, PhD, RD

Acknowledgments

Special thanks to Reed Mangels, PhD, RD; Cathy Conway, MS, RD; and VRG dietetic intern Erin M. Crandell for reviewing the contents of this book and contributing content. Thanks to Meri Robie for the preliminary editing and layout for this book, and to David Herring, MS, and Susan Petrie for proofreading the entire manuscript. Finally, thanks to Keryl Cryer for designing the cover and doing all the artwork and Debra Wasserman for coordinating all aspects of this book's production from start to finish, including final layout preparations. Your help is greatly appreciated.

Introduction

THIS VEGAN DIABETIC MENU PLANNER is designed to provide followers with a balance of protein, carbohydrates, fat, vitamins, and minerals while following the basic principles of a diabetic meal plan. Since every person with diabetes has his or her own individual energy and nutrient needs, please consult your health care professional to make sure our suggestions will work for you. Note: The menu planner is designed for young adults through seniors. It is <u>not</u> designed for children or people who need close medical management of diabetes.

The menus have been written based on the American Diabetes Association's Exchange Lists for Meal Planning. Since carbohydrates are the nutrients that diabetics need to monitor the closest, the exchange lists are designed to help maintain the proper amount of carbohydrates in your diet. Carbohydrates, proteins, and fats are the three major nutrients found in the foods we eat, but carbohydrates have the greatest effect on our blood sugar. Since controlling blood sugar is the number one goal of diabetes management, controlling your intake of carbohydrates can help you achieve that goal. This doesn't mean that carbohydrates should be eliminated; rather, it becomes important for you to plan your meals and snacks so they provide a consistent amount of carbohydrates. And that brings us back to the Exchange Lists.

The Exchange Lists include foods from the following food groups: Starches, Fruit, Milk, Vegetables, Proteins, Fats, and "Free Foods." Carbohydrates are primarily found in the Starches, Fruit, and Milk groups. One serving (or exchange) of a Starch, Fruit, or Milk will provide 15 grams of carbohydrates (the amount of protein and fat in each carbohydrate exchange will vary, depending on the food). Monitoring serving sizes in this way is also referred to as "carbohydrate counting."

For example, your breakfast meal may allow three servings of carbohydrates, or 45 grams of carbohydrates. The three servings can be distributed among different foods—maybe two Starches and one Fruit. A snack may allow two servings of carbohydrates, or 30 grams. In this case, one Milk and one Starch would work well. Just remember that Starches, Fruits, and Milk provide carbohydrates, and one serving of carbohydrates provides 15 grams.

Vegetables, proteins, and fats usually provide little carbohydrates, but are good sources of other important nutrients, namely vitamins and minerals. In general, vegetables contain only a few grams of carbohydrates (5 grams per serving) and can be used more liberally in the diabetic diet. In some cases they are not included in carbohydrate counting. As such, we have not counted them in these menus. However your health professional may recommend that you include the carbohydrate count of these vegetables in your meal planning. Also, if you eat very large quantities of these vegetables (i.e., several cups), they should be counted as a carbohydrate serving. Starchy vegetables—corn, peas, lima beans, potatoes, sweet potatoes, and winter squash—must be counted as a carbohydrate serving. They are considered a Starch and contain 15 grams of carbohydrates per serving. Proteins and fats are an important part of any diet, and actually work well with carbohydrates to help stabilize blood sugar. One protein exchange equals one ounce of "meat." One fat exchange equals five grams of fat.

Trying to digest all of this information can be difficult! Feel free to obtain your own copy of the Exchange Lists by calling the American Diabetes Association at (800) 232-3472, or visit them online at <WWW.DIABETES.ORG>. The American Dietetic Association also provides helpful information on meal planning for diabetes. Visit <WWW.EATRIGHT.ORG>.

Vegan Menu for People with Diabetes

Exchanges and Their Equivalents

Each exchange provides the following:

1 **starch** (bread) exchange = 80 calories;
15 grams carbohydrates

*(e.g., 1 slice bread, 1/2 English muffin or bagel, 1/2 cup hot cooked cereal,
1 tortilla, 1/3 cup cooked rice, 1/2 cup cooked pasta,
1/2 cup starchy vegetable)*

1 **fruit** exchange = 60 calories;
15 grams carbohydrates

*(e.g., 1 small piece fresh fruit, 1/2 cup water- or juice-packed canned or
frozen fruit, 2 Tablespoons dried fruit, 1/2 cup fruit juice)*

1 **milk** exchange = 120 calories;
12 grams carbohydrates

(e.g., 8 ounces enriched soymilk)

1 **vegetable** exchange = 25 calories;
5 grams carbohydrates

(e.g., 1/2 cup cooked, 1 cup raw, 1/2 cup vegetable juice)

1 **very lean protein** exchange = 35 calories;
1 **lean protein** exchange = 55 calories;
1 **high-fat protein** exchange = 100 calories;
0 grams carbohydrates

(e.g., 1/2 cup or 4 ounces tofu, 1/2 cup cooked beans,
2 Tablespoons nut butters, 2 ounces meat substitutes)*

*Because of the carbohydrate content in beans, 1/2 cup must also be considered 1 starch.

1 **fat** exchange = 45 calories;
0 grams carbohydrates

*(e.g., 1 Tablespoon regular salad dressing, 2 Tablespoons reduced-fat
salad dressing, 1-1/2 Tablespoons vegan mayonnaise)*

Nutritionally, the daily menu breaks down to approximately 1800 calories per day, 50% of these from carbohydrates, 20% from protein, and 30% from fat.

Daily Menu Pattern

Each daily menu follows the pattern below. If followed closely, the meal plan provides approximately 1800 calories per day. The amount of carbohydrates (CHO) at each meal has been calculated:

Breakfast: 385 calories
1 fruit	15 grams CHO
2 starch	30 grams CHO
1 fat	
1 milk	15 grams CHO

Morning Snack: 140 calories
1 starch	15 grams CHO
1 fruit	15 grams CHO

Lunch: 420 calories
2 starch	30 grams CHO
2 fat	
1 vegetable	
1 protein	
1 milk	15 grams CHO

Afternoon Snack: 155 calories
1 starch	15 grams CHO
1 protein	

Dinner: 560 calories
2 protein	
1 fat	
1 vegetable	
2 starch	30 grams CHO
1 fruit	15 grams CHO
1 milk	15 grams CHO

Evening Snack: 155 calories
1 starch	15 grams CHO
1 protein	

Total: 1815 calories

This may be a lot of information for you at first! Begin to use the menus, and you will become proficient in figuring out how many exchanges you are eating. Once you know the exchanges, you can easily figure out the calories and amount of carbs you are eating daily.

Vegan Menu for People with Diabetes

How To Use the Menus

These menus were planned with a great deal of variety so as to be appealing. We realize that it may not be practical for you to include such a wide assortment of foods at all times, due to preparation time, busy schedules, seasonal limitations on fresh vegetables, and other reasons.

Keeping in mind that a varied diet is necessary for good nutrition—you can still repeat some of your favorite days and exclude several of your least favorite days. You can also use menu days out of sequence, depending on your shopping and cooking schedule. However, be sure to use a whole day of menus, as each day has been balanced for good nutrition, calories, vitamins, and other considerations.

What to do with the inevitable leftovers? If you have a whole snack or entrée left over, refrigerate it properly, and skip a day before eating it. Even better, freeze it so you can eat it again when you're ready for it. It's not a good idea to eat the same foods several days in a row, as you'll cheat yourself of optimal nutrition.

You will probably need to invest in a small portion scale and a set of measuring cups and spoons. After a while, you will become adept at correct portion sizes. Remember, the amount of food you eat is just as important as the type of food.

The menus were designed to require less preparation on working days (Monday through Friday) and for lunches. It's probably a good idea to prepare work or school day lunches and snacks the night before so you can grab them and go. You might want to invest in some insulated carrying bags and cups so you can transport your food safely.

Saturday and Sunday menus intentionally require a little more food preparation. Use these days whenever your "off" days occur, so you'll have time to prepare your meals and enjoy.

You'll notice that the menus are designed as six small meals a day. Eating in this way better stabilizes your blood sugar, providing a steady influx of energy and helping you feel well.

You may find that you can purchase some of the meals and snacks, rather than packing them. That's fine; just watch portion sizes and "extras" such as oil added to popped corn, protein powder added to smoothies, and other hidden calories.

If you need to eat fewer calories than the menus offer, first reduce the starch (pasta, potatoes, popcorn, etc.) exchanges. One serving of starch, equivalent to one slice of bread or 1/2 cup cooked pasta, is approximately 80 calories. However, before you change your dietary pattern, be certain to consult your dietitian or health care professional. A dietary change may require a change in medication or monitoring.

These menus are moderate in fat. If you require an adjustment in the fat levels, consult with your health care professional. If you follow the menus exactly and make no non-vegan substitutions, then there will be no cholesterol in your diet. Foods high in saturated fat or trans fatty acids should be avoided, if possible. Read food labels and try to stay away from foods containing palm oil, coconut oil, other tropical oils, and hydrogenated vegetable fat.

Most of the recipes found on these menus are taken from *Vegan Meals for One or Two*. The number besides the recipe title in the menu is the page where the recipe can be found in this book. Additionally, each recipe indicates the pages where it is called for in the menu. There is a designation on the menus as to how much of each recipe is considered a portion. Don't assume that the recipe always makes the portion size called for in the menu. For example, the recipe for Corn and Potato Chowder makes three servings. The menu beside it lists:

1 serving **Corn and Potato Chowder**

Therefore, divide the chowder into three equal portions and freeze the rest, or make only one-third of the recipe. The amount listed in the daily menu will keep you on the correct daily exchange pattern. With menu items that do not have a recipe, we've included additional preparation information if necessary.

Before heading off to the kitchen, take a look at the four weeks of menus we've suggested. Let your health care professional take a look at them, too, to see if they need to be personalized for you. Spend some time reviewing the ingredients and the recipes, making shopping lists, and scheduling meal preparation.

It takes effort to live well with diabetes. Controlling this disease may be a lot of work; but living a long, healthy life will be worth it!

Food Selection and Preparation Guidelines

1. When sautéeing or cooking food in a skillet, use a minimum of vegetable oil spray, rather than cooking oil or margarine.

2. If you use margarine, look for brands that contain few or no trans fatty acids.

3. Purchase enriched soymilk, looking for brands that have vitamins B_{12} and D, and calcium.

4. Purchase tofu processed with calcium. You can find this information on the label of packaged tofu. If purchasing freshly made tofu, ask the manufacturer about its content.

5. Red Star™ Nutritional Yeast (Vegetarian Support Formula) is a good source of vegan vitamin B_{12}. The yeast can be sprinkled on cereals, rice, soups, vegetables, pasta, and entrées. Use 1 to 2 teaspoons per serving.

6. All foods must be weighed or measured. Invest in a small kitchen or portion scale. Make sure you have a set of measuring cups and spoons handy. When storing leftover prepared food, you might want to measure it out in portion sizes before you package it. This will make meal time preparation go faster.

Free Foods

Some items are so low in calories and fat that they are considered "free." You may add these to your meal preparations as you like. Here is a list of some foods that are considered "free":

Fat-free and sodium-free broth (use this as a cooking liquid for vegetables and grains, or chop some fresh veggies into broth and use as a fast no-calorie snack)

Sparkling water and seltzers (with a squeeze of lemon or lime, these make a good "hydration" break)

Unsweetened cocoa powder (add 1 Tablespoon to pudding mixes, hot cereals, or soymilk)

Unsweetened fresh or frozen cranberries and rhubarb (these are very sour—chop and use sparingly in fat-free salad dressings; cook with rice, barley, or couscous; or add to fresh salads)

Mustard, horseradish, catsup (1 Tablespoon), **vinegar**

Unsweetened pickled vegetables: okra, cucumbers, carrots, cauliflower, etc. (Although there is no limit on these, if you are on a sodium restriction, try and have no more than a couple of Tablespoons of these per day.)

Fat-free, low-calorie salad dressing

1 cup raw vegetables: cabbage, celery, cucumber, green onion, garlic, hot peppers and chilies, mushrooms, radishes, summer squash (you can make a great "extra" salad or relish by combining a mixture of these veggies with some vinegar or non-fat salad dressing)

Greens: up to 4 cups of fresh endive, raddichio, chicory, head lettuces, romaine, spinach, kale, chard, mustard greens, and beet greens per day

Vegan Menu for People with Diabetes

Learning to Read a Label

For convenience, you may at times want to use some prepared products. Learning to read a food label is essential. Each packaged food has a nutrition label listing the number of carbohydrates per serving. When reading a nutrition label, look for the total carbohydrates. Many packages contain two or more servings. It's important to check how many servings are in a package. If you eat a package of food that contains two servings of carbohydrates, your intake will be twice the amount of total carbohydrates listed on the label. Use the label below to test yourself!

Question: If you eat 2 cups of this food, how many grams of carbohydrates are you having?

Nutrition Facts

Serving Size 1 cup (228 g)
Servings per Container 2

Amount per serving

Calories 90
Calories from fat 30

	% Daily Values
Total Fat 3g	5%
Saturated fat 0g	0%
Cholesterol 0mg	0%
Sodium 300mg	13%
Total Carbohydrate 13g	4%
Dietary Fiber 3g	12%
Sugars 3g	
Protein 3g	

←Be aware of the serving size and number of servings!

←Look for total grams of carbohydrate, not just sugars!

Answer: 26g

Spice Up That Soymilk!

SOME PEOPLE really enjoy soymilk and drinking eight ounces of soymilk at each meal will be no problem. If it's a new food to you, though, some adjustment may be necessary.

Here, variety is the spice of life. You can flavor your soymilk with any ingredient that does not add calories. That means you could add favorites, such as vanilla, orange, rum, almond, and lemon extracts. If you have time and plan ahead, you can flavor your soymilk for the next meal and freeze it to enjoy a soy slushie that can be a refreshing beverage or a frozen dessert. Make a low-cal hot cocoa by adding unsweetened cocoa powder to warm soymilk. Indulge yourself and make some soymilk lattes or Indian spiced tea with soymilk.

You can use the soymilk to be consumed with each meal in cooking that meal. For example, you might want to add a small portion of your meal's soymilk to a tomato soup to make it "creamy," or add some soymilk to a mushroom sauce.

There are commercially flavored soymilks on the market, such as chocolate, mocha, and vanilla. Do a label comparison. If the nutritional profile is the same as for plain soymilk, you can alternate flavored milks.

Menus
and
Recipes

Corny French Toast
(Makes 3 slices)

2 Tablespoons silken tofu
1/4 cup vanilla soy or rice milk
1/4 teaspoon nutmeg
1/2 teaspoon cinnamon
1 cup cornflakes
3 slices whole wheat or raisin bread
Vegetable oil spray

In a bowl, combine tofu, milk, nutmeg, and cinnamon until smooth.

Crumble cornflakes (you're not looking for cornflake flour; crumble until each flake is broken in two or three pieces). Spread flakes on a dinner plate.

Dip bread in the tofu mixture until both sides are coated. Place each slice of bread (both sides) into the cornflakes. Press down slightly so they stick. Spray frying pan with vegetable oil and fry bread until each side is golden brown.

Serve with sliced bananas, fruit preserves, or syrup.

Note: If you don't have vanilla flavored soy or rice milk, use plain, and add a half teaspoon of vanilla extract and a quarter teaspoon sweetener. Also, if you're not a fan of frying (or you want to have breakfast cooking while you do other things), you can bake this recipe. Preheat oven to 375 degrees while you prepare the bread. Spray a baking sheet with vegetable oil and place the prepared bread on it. Bake for approximately 20 minutes or until golden and puffy.

Total calories per 1 slice serving, using soymilk and whole wheat bread: 385

Total Fat as % of Daily Value: 11%	**Dietary Fiber: 7 g**
Protein: 13 g	**Fat: 7 g**
Carbohydrates: 69 g	**Calcium: 107 mg**
Iron: 4 mg	**Sodium: 716 mg**

Exchange: 2 slices = 3 starch and 1 fat

Sunday: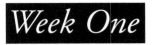

Breakfast:
1/2 cup melon slices
2 slices **Corny French Toast** (page 18) with
1/4 cup chopped peaches or apricots
4 ounces enriched soymilk

Morning Snack:
1/2 cup fresh grapes
6 assorted lowfat crackers
Sparkling water

Lunch:
1 cup mushroom barley soup** with
2 ounces smoked seitan* See glossary.
1/2 cup green and wax bean salad
with 2 teaspoons sesame seeds
and 2 Tablespoons reduced-fat salad dressing
8 ounces enriched soymilk

Afternoon Snack:
1/2 cup sugar-free chocolate pudding*
See glossary.

Dinner:
1 cup **Lentil Chili** (page 20)
with 1/4 cup prepared TVP* See glossary.
over 1/3 cup white rice
1/2 cup steamed or roasted carrots
1/2 cup fresh pineapple slices

Evening Snack:
1/2 cup pretzels
8 ounces enriched soymilk

**Try Tabatchnik's, Hains, or Healthy Choice vegan soups.

Lentil Chili

(Makes 1 portion)

this recipe is used on page 19

1/2 cup drained canned or cooked lentils
1/4 cup chopped tomatoes
1/4 cup prepared salsa
1/2 teaspoon red pepper flakes
1/2 teaspoon chili powder

Combine all ingredients and stir to mix. Microwave, covered, for 4 minutes on HIGH, or cook on stove in a small pot until heated through.

Total calories per serving: 153
Total Fat as % of Daily Value: 2%
Protein: 11 g
Carbohydrates: 28 g
Iron: 4 mg

Dietary Fiber: 10 g
Fat: 1 g
Calcium: 45 mg
Sodium: 300 mg

Exchange: 2 Starch + 1 Vegetable + 1 Very Lean Protein

Monday: Week One

Breakfast:
1/3 cup cranberry juice or cranberry juice cocktail
3/4 cup cooked oatmeal with 1/2 banana
and 1 teaspoon vegan margarine
8 ounces enriched soymilk

Morning Snack:
3 cups lowfat popped popcorn
sprinkled with 2 teaspoons nutritional yeast
1/2 cup orange juice

Lunch:
6-inch pita stuffed with
2 ounces fake meat* See glossary.
(equivalent to 2 ADA meat exchanges)
lettuce, radishes, cucumbers, and
1 cup shredded cabbage
mixed with 1-1/2 Tablespoons vegan mayonnaise
8 ounces enriched soymilk

Afternoon Snack:
Fruit Smoothie: made with
8 ounces enriched soymilk, 2 ounces silken tofu,
and 1/2 cup frozen or fresh berries, blended together
3 ginger snaps

Dinner:
Baked eggplant (1/2 cup) with 1/4 cup tomato sauce
1/2 cup black beans with 1/3 cup brown rice
1 medium baked apple

Evening Snack:
2 Tablespoons peanut butter on
6 crackers

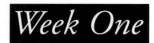 **Tuesday:**

Breakfast:
1/2 cup orange slices
2 slices whole wheat toast spread with
2 Tablespoons peanut butter
8 ounces enriched soymilk

Morning Snack:
5 vanilla wafers
1/2 cup apricot nectar

Lunch:
1-1/2 cups spinach and Romaine salad
with fat-free salad dressing,
1 Tablespoon sliced berries, and 6 almonds
Bean Enchilada: fold 1/2 cup beans
into 1 tortilla and top with salsa
8 ounces enriched soymilk

Afternoon Snack:
1/2 cup soy ice cream

Dinner:
1/2 cup steamed broccoli
with 1/4 cup red peppers
1 cup steamed, baked, roasted,
or microwaved potatoes
seasoned with 1/2 teaspoon curry powder
and 2 Tablespoons vegan sour cream
1 veggie hot dog or 1 ounce vegan deli slices

Evening Snack:
3 graham crackers with 2 Tablespoons nut butter
8 ounces enriched soymilk

Vegan Menu for People with Diabetes

Wednesday: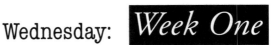

Breakfast:
1/2 cup apricot nectar
Breakfast Pizza: 2 English muffin halves spread with
1 teaspoon vegan margarine and
1-1/2 ounces vegan soy cheese
topped with 1/2 cup salsa
8 ounces enriched soymilk

Morning Snack:
1/2 cup fat-free tortilla or pita chips
1/2 cup carrot juice

Lunch:
1 cup vegetable bean soup**
1/4 bagel spread with 2 teaspoons soy cream cheese
1/4 bagel with 1 Tablespoon nut butter
8 ounces enriched soymilk

Afternoon Snack:
Creamy Tomato Smoothie: made with
1 cup tomato juice and 1/2 cup silken tofu

Dinner:
6 ounce grilled portobello mushroom "steak"
1/2 cup braised swiss chard
1/2 cup baked or steamed sweet potato
topped with 2 Tablespoons canned pineapple chunks
1/2 cup baked tofu

Evening Snack:
1 medium pear or apple
8 ounces enriched soymilk

**Try Tabachnik's or Healthy Choice vegan soups, or prepare
your own from scratch!

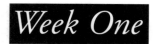

Thursday:

Breakfast:
1/4 cup cranberry apple juice
1 cup hot whole grain cereal mixed with
1/4 cup peaches and 1 teaspoon vegan margarine
8 ounces enriched soymilk

Morning Snack:
1/2 cup vegetable juice (V-8, for example)
1 cup croutons or crackers

Lunch:
Veggie Wrap:
One 7- to 8-inch tortilla with 1/2 cup grilled vegetables,
1-1/2 Tablespoons vegan mayonnaise,
1-1/2 ounces vegan cheese, and 6 strips vegan bacon
8 ounces enriched soymilk

Afternoon Snack:
1/2 cup baked veggie chips with
1/2 cup non-fat refried beans mixed with salsa

Dinner:
8 ounces baked tofu with 1/4 cup tomato sauce
1/2 cup steamed spinach and onions
1 dinner roll spread with 1 teaspoon vegan margarine
1/2 cup grapes

Evening Snack:
3 cups lowfat popcorn
sprinkled with 2 teaspoons nutritional yeast
8 ounces enriched soymilk

Friday: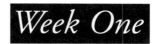

Breakfast:
1/2 cup cold whole grain cereal topped
with 1/2 cup sliced banana
1 slice toast spread with 1 teaspoon vegan margarine
8 ounces enriched soymilk

Morning Snack:
1 medium fresh apple or pear
2 breadsticks

Lunch:
2 veggie burgers on 1/2 whole wheat bun
layered with lettuce, tomato, and shredded carrots
Cucumber sticks
8 ounces enriched soymilk

Afternoon Snack:
1/2 cup sugar-free vanilla pudding* See glossary.
with 2 Tablespoons pistachios or pecans

Dinner:
1 cup pasta with *Mushroom Sauce:* use
1/2 cup soymilk, 1/4 cup minced mushrooms,
and 1 teaspoon garlic—heat and add 2 chunks tofu
1/2 cup braised kale or chard
1 cup berries
4 ounces enriched soymilk

Evening Snack:
2 Tablespoons nut butter
with 3 ginger snaps

Corn and Potato Chowder
(Makes 3 servings)

Vegetable oil spray
1/2 cup chopped onions
2 minced garlic cloves
1/8 cup chopped fresh parsley
1-1/4 cups frozen cut corn, thawed, or corn cut from
   3 ears of corn
3 cups water
4 cubed boiling potatoes
1 teaspoon dried dill
2 cups soymilk
1 cup silken tofu
1 teaspoon thyme
1/2 teaspoon black pepper

In a large pot, spray vegetable oil and heat. Add onions, garlic, parsley, and corn. Cover the pot and simmer for 20 minutes, stirring frequently. Add water and bring to a boil. Add potatoes and simmer, uncovered, until potatoes are tender, approximately 30 minutes.

   Stir in dill, soymilk, tofu, thyme, and pepper. Simmer chowder for 15 minutes or until very hot.

Total calories per serving: 309
Total Fat as % of Daily Value: 10%   Dietary Fiber: 8 g
Protein: 15 g   Fat: 7 g
Carbohydrates: 53 g   Calcium: 75 mg
Iron: 4 mg   Sodium: 39mg
Exchange: 2 protein + 1 vegetable + 2 starch

Saturday:

Breakfast:
1 cup melon or mango slices
Breakfast Soft Tacos:
2 tortillas with 2 teaspoons vegan margarine
and 1/2 cup salsa
8 ounces enriched soymilk

Morning Snack:
1/2 cup pineapple slices
1/4 cup fat-free granola

Lunch:
1 cup scrambled tofu with chopped veggies
1/2 English muffin
1 medium ear of corn
with 1 teaspoon vegan margarine
8 ounces enriched soymilk

Afternoon Snack:
1/2 cup red bean chili with 2 ounces tofu

Dinner:
1 serving **Corn and Potato Chowder** (page 26)
with 1/2 cup tofu added
1/2 cup tomato wedges
1 cup berries

Evening Snack:
1/2 cup soy ice cream
sprinkled with 2 Tablespoons granola

Cinnamon, Apple, and Raisin Pancakes
(Makes about 4 six-inch pancakes)

1-1/2 cups all-purpose flour
1/4 cup vegan dry sweetener* See glossary.
2 teaspoons baking powder
2 teaspoons cinnamon
1 cup plain or vanilla soymilk
2 Tablespoons silken tofu
1 Tablespoon oil or melted vegan margarine
1/4 teaspoon vanilla extract
Vegetable oil spray
2 large green apples (about 1 cup), peeled, cored,
  and minced
1/2 cup raisins

Sift flour, sweetener, baking powder, and cinnamon and place in a large bowl. In a separate bowl, mix soymilk, tofu, oil or vegan margarine, and vanilla together until well combined. Slowly mix dry and liquid ingredients together until smooth. Cover and refrigerate for at least 1 hour.

Heat a large frying pan and spray with oil. Add apples and raisins and sauté for 3 minutes or until apples begin to soften. Place in a bowl and set aside.

Respray pan and ladle batter into the pan by 1/2 cup measures. Top each with 2 Tablespoons of apple/raisin mixture. Cook until pancakes begin to bubble. Flip and cook until golden brown.

Note: This batter can be prepared the night before and left in the refrigerator overnight.

Total calories per pancake using plain soymilk: 393

Total Fat as % of Daily Value: 9%	**Dietary Fiber: 5 g**
Protein: 15 g	**Fat: 6 g**
Carbohydrates: 76 g	**Calcium: 175 mg**
Iron: 4 mg	**Sodium: 256 mg**

Exchange: 3 Starch + 1 Fruit + 1 Fat

Vegan Menu for People with Diabetes

Breakfast:
1/2 cup red grapefruit sections, broiled
or 1/2 fresh grapefruit
1 **Cinnamon, Apple, and Raisin Pancake** (page 28)
8 ounces enriched soymilk

Morning Snack:
1 small baked apple
topped with 3 teaspoons granola

Lunch:
1 cup steamed broccoli, red pepper, and cauliflower
mixed with 1/2 cup black beans and
1/4 cup prepared TVP
over 1/3 cup rice or barley
1/2 cup spinach salad with 1/4 cup raspberries
8 ounces enriched soymilk

Afternoon Snack:
Waldorf Salad: 3/4 cup chopped apple,
1/4 cup celery, 1 Tablespoon walnuts, and
1-1/2 Tablespoons vegan mayonnaise

Dinner:
2 slices veggie pizza
Chopped Romaine lettuce with fat-free dressing

Evening Snack:
1/2 cup pretzels
8 ounces enriched soymilk

Baked Pasta and Peppers
(Makes 3 servings)

Vegetable oil spray
1/2 cup cooked orzo, pastina, or other small-shaped
  pasta
1/2 cup shredded vegan soy cheese
1/4 cup diced red bell pepper
1/4 cup sliced canned mushrooms, drained
1/2 cup soy sour cream* See glossary.
1 teaspoon pepper
1/2 teaspoon granulated garlic
1/2 teaspoon onion powder
1 Tablespoon vegan margarine

Preheat oven to 400 degrees. Spray a 1-quart (small) baking dish with oil. Combine all ingredients, except margarine, in a baking dish. Dot with margarine. Bake approximately 15 minutes, uncovered, until golden.

Note: Orzo and pastina are very small pasta shapes, almost resembling rice or grains. They cook very nicely and can be used for savory dishes, like this one, or even instead of hot cereal, in the morning.

Total calories per serving: 114
Total Fat as % of Daily Value: 9%   Dietary Fiber: 1 g
Protein: 5 g   Fat: 8 g
Carbohydrates: 12 g   Calcium: 46 mg
Iron: 1 mg   Sodium: 121 mg
Exchange: 1 Protein + 1/2 Vegetable + 1 Starch + 1 Fat
(Note: This is for 1 serving. The Meal Plan is for 2 servings.)

Monday: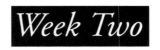

Breakfast:
1/2 cup orange juice
3/4 cup whole wheat cold cereal and
1/4 cup fat-free granola
8 ounces enriched soymilk

Morning Snack:
1/2 cup apricot nectar
5 vanilla wafers

Lunch:
Mixed Bean Burrito:
fold 1 tortilla around 3/4 cup beans
(black, navy, pinto) with salsa
1 cup Romaine salad
with 2 Tablespoons Kalamata or green olives
and 1 Tablespoon reduced-fat dressing
8 ounces enriched soymilk

Afternoon Snack:
3/4 cup 3-bean salad (garbanzo, wax, green)
with fat-free dressing

Dinner:
2 servings **Baked Pasta and Peppers** (page 30)
Baked pear

Evening Snack:
1-1/2 Tablespoons soy nuts
2 breadsticks with 2 Tablespoons hummus
8 ounces enriched soymilk

Wonder Gazpacho

(Makes 2 servings)

1 cup chopped, ripe tomatoes
2 Tablespoons tomato paste
1/8 cup chopped cucumbers
1/4 cup chopped bell peppers
1/8 cup chopped onions
1 minced garlic clove or 1 teaspoon granulated garlic
1 teaspoon cracked black pepper
2 teaspoons lemon or lime juice

Place all the ingredients in a blender and pulse until a chunky texture is achieved. Pour into serving bowls and chill for at least 30 minutes before serving.

Note: This cold soup can be made spicier by adding salsa or chopped chilies.

Total calories per serving: 48
Total Fat as % of Daily Value: <1%   **Dietary Fiber: 3 g**
Protein: 2 g   **Fat: <1 g**
Carbohydrates: 11 g   **Calcium: 23 mg**
Iron: 1 mg   **Sodium: 24 mg**
Exchange: 1 Fruit

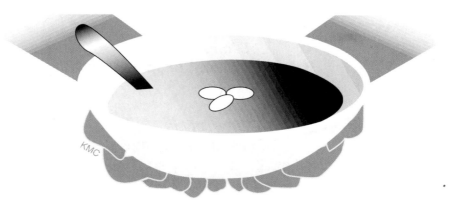

Vegan Menu for People with Diabetes

Tuesday: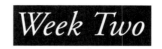

Breakfast:
1/3 cup cranberry juice cocktail
3/4 cup **Apple Oatmeal** (page 34)
8 ounces enriched soymilk

Morning Snack:
1 small banana
2 rice cakes

Lunch:
1 serving **Wonder Gazpacho** (page 32)
4 whole wheat crackers
1/2 cup *Carrot and Raisin Salad:* 1/2 cup carrots,
2 teaspoons vegan mayonnaise, and 1 teaspoon raisins
8 ounces enriched soymilk

Afternoon Snack:
1/2 cup fruit-flavored soy yogurt

Dinner:
1 serving **Tofu Scramble** (page 34)
1/2 cup braised chard
4 ounces sugar-free chocolate pudding
with 2 Tablespoons berries

Evening Snack:
1/2 cup baked sweet potatoes
topped with 2 teaspoons soy cream cheese
8 ounces enriched soymilk

Apple Oatmeal
(Makes 1-1/2 cups)

this recipe is used on page 33

1 small apple, cored and chopped
1/2 cup apple juice
1 teaspoon cinnamon
2/3 cup rolled oats (oatmeal)
1/4 cup chopped walnuts

In a medium-sized pot, combine all the ingredients and bring to a fast boil. Reduce heat and simmer, stirring for 5 minutes or until oatmeal is cooked to the texture you like.

Total calories per 3/4 cup serving: 258
Total Fat as % of Daily Value: 17%   **Dietary Fiber: 5.5 g**
Protein: 6.5 g   **Fat: 11 g**
Carbohydrates: 36 g   **Calcium: 50 mg**
Iron: 2 mg   **Sodium: 4 mg**
Exchange: 2 Starch + 2 Fat

Tofu Scramble
(Makes 1 hearty serving)

this recipe is used on page 33

1 cup plain firm tofu, drained and crumbled
Vegetable oil spray
1/4 cup chopped leftover veggies
2 Tablespoons salsa

In a small bowl, mash tofu. Heat a small frying pan and spray with oil. Place tofu in the pan and mix in veggies. Stir and sauté until the veggies are soft and the tofu is heated through. Mix in the salsa and allow scramble to cook until heated. Serve hot.

Total calories per serving, using chopped green peppers and onions: 395
Total Fat as % of Daily Value: 35%   **Dietary Fiber: 7 g**

Vegan Menu for People with Diabetes

Protein: 41 g
Carbohydrates: 15 g
Iron: 27 mg
Exchange: 5 Protein + 1 Starch

Fat: 23 g
Calcium: 429 mg
Sodium: 120 mg

Power Chili
(Makes 4 servings)

this recipe is used on page 37

Vegetable oil spray
2 minced garlic cloves
1/2 cup diced onions
1/4 cup diced green bell pepper
1/4 cup diced red bell pepper
1/2 cup soy sausage (Soyrizo is good, as are other kinds
   of smoky-flavored vegan sausage)
1/2 cup frozen cut corn, thawed
1-1/2 cups cooked beans, drained (canned are fine;
   use different varieties)
1 cup vegetable broth
2 teaspoons chili powder
1 teaspoon red pepper flakes
1/2 teaspoon cumin

Heat a large pot and spray with oil. Add garlic, onions, and peppers and sauté until soft. Add sausage and sauté until cooked, approximately 3 minutes. Be sure to crumble sausage. Add remaining ingredients and bring to a fast boil. Reduce heat, allow to simmer until veggies are tender, approximately 30 minutes. The longer this chili cooks, the more flavorful it becomes. Serve warm or freeze for later use.

Total calories per serving, using red kidney beans: 174
Total Fat as % of Daily Value: 4%   Dietary Fiber: 11 g
Protein: 3 g   Fat: 3 g
Carbohydrates: 31 g   Calcium: 20 mg
Iron: 1 mg   Sodium: 351 mg
Exchange: 1 Starch + 2 Protein

Tangy Tofu Salad
(1 hearty serving or 2 average servings)

1 Tablespoon olive oil
1/8 cup red wine or balsamic vinegar
1/2 teaspoon dried basil
1/4 teaspoon black pepper
1/4 teaspoon dried oregano
8 ounces firm tofu, cut into medium-sized cubes
3 or 4 lettuce leaves or 1 cup pre-cut salad mix
2 or 3 tomato slices
2 Tablespoons diced onion

In a medium-sized bowl, combine oil, vinegar, basil, pepper, and oregano. Toss well. Add tofu, then place in a refrigerator and allow to sit for 15 minutes.

In a salad bowl, combine lettuce, tomatoes, and onions. Add tofu mixture and toss before serving.

Total calories per 1 hearty serving: 253
Total Fat as % of Daily Value: 26%   Dietary Fiber: 4 g
Protein: 19 g   Fat: 17 g
Carbohydrates: 9 g   Calcium: 220 mg
Iron: 13 mg   Sodium: 27 mg
Exchange: 2 Protein + 1 Vegetable + 1 Fat

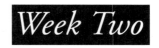

Wednesday:

Breakfast:
1/4 cup apricot nectar
3/4 cup cold whole grain cereal topped with
1/4 cup banana
1 slice toast, spread with 1 teaspoon vegan margarine
8 ounces enriched soymilk

Morning Snack:
1 cup fresh or frozen berries
1/2 cup pretzels

Lunch:
1 serving **Power Chili** (page 35)
over cornbread (2x3-inch)
spread with 1 teaspoon vegan margarine
Cucumber sticks
8 ounces enriched soymilk

Afternoon Snack:
Fruit Smoothie: made with 1/4 cup soy yogurt,
3/4 cup enriched soymilk, 2 Tablespoons banana,
and 2 teaspoons orange juice concentrate

Dinner:
1 hearty serving **Tangy Tofu Salad** (page 36)
1/2 cup seasonal fruit salad
4 breadsticks

Evening Snack:
3 graham crackers
8 ounces enriched soymilk

Pasta in Paradise
(Makes 2 servings)

4 ounces uncooked vermicelli, rice noodles, or
  spaghetti
1/4 cup red or yellow bell pepper strips (about 1
  medium pepper)
1 cup ripe chopped papaya (about 1 small papaya)
1 cup ripe chopped tomatoes (about 1 medium tomato)
1/2 cup ripe, chopped mango (about 1/2 mango)
2 Tablespoons chopped fresh cilantro or flat-leafed
  parsley
2 teaspoons olive oil
1/4 teaspoon cinnamon
1/2 teaspoon white pepper
2 Tablespoons chopped peanuts

Cook pasta according to package directions. Rinse, drain,
and set aside to cool. In a large bowl, combine pepper,
papaya, tomatoes, mango, cilantro, oil, cinnamon, and
white pepper and toss to mix. Add pasta and toss to mix.
Top with peanuts.

Total calories per serving, using rice noodles and cilantro: 376
Total Fat as % of Daily Value: 15%   Dietary Fiber: 4 g
Protein: 7 g   Fat: 10 g
Carbohydrates: 68 g   Calcium: 44 mg
Iron: 2 mg   Sodium: 19 mg
Exchange: 1 Protein + 1 Fat + 4 Starch

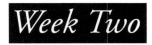

Thursday:

Breakfast:
1/4 cup pineapple and 1/4 cup orange juice, blended
Breakfast Parfait: made with 6 ounces soy yogurt,
1/4 cup berries, and 1/4 cup granola
4 ounces enriched soymilk

Morning Snack:
1/2 cup fresh grapes or sliced papaya

Lunch:
1 serving **Pasta in Paradise** (page 38)
1/2 cup shredded red and green cabbage
mixed with 2 Tablespoons hummus
4 ounces enriched soymilk

Afternoon Snack:
2 Tablespoons peanut butter
4 crackers

Dinner:
1-1/2 servings **Salsa Black Bean Salad** (page 41)
1/3 cup brown rice
1/2 cup melon

Evening Snack:
1 pita
4 ounces enriched soymilk

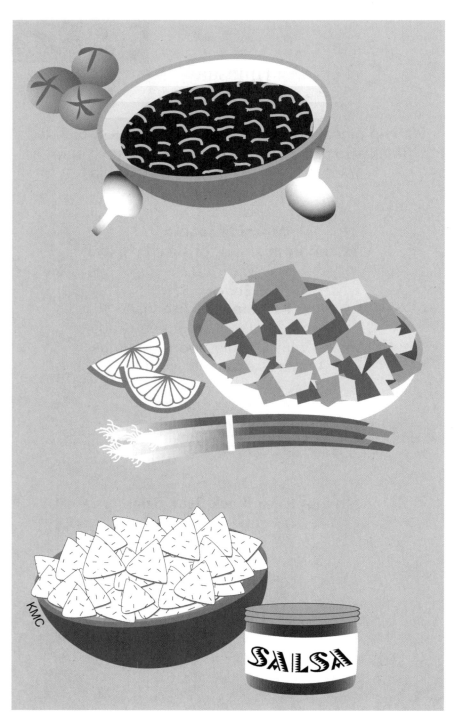

Salsa Black Bean Salad
(Makes 2 servings)

this recipe is used on page 39

1 cup cooked black beans (if canned, drain and rinse)
1/2 fresh orange, peeled and chopped
1/8 cup chopped green onions
1/4 cup salsa
1 Tablespoon lemon or lime juice
1 minced garlic clove or 1 teaspoon granulated garlic
1 teaspoon cumin
1 teaspoon red pepper flakes
Shredded lettuce, as desired
Tortilla chips or shredded tortillas, as desired

Mix beans, oranges, onions, salsa, juice, garlic, cumin, and pepper flakes together in a medium bowl. Chill for at least 1 hour. Serve over lettuce and garnish with chips.

Total calories per serving, using lemon juice, but without lettuce or chips: 158

Total Fat as % of Daily Value: 2%	Dietary Fiber: 10 g
Protein: 9 g	Fat: 1 g
Carbohydrates: 30 g	Calcium: 75 mg
Iron: 3 mg	Sodium: 88 mg

Exchange: 1 Protein + 1 Vegetable + 1 Starch

Stuffed Peppers
(Makes 4 peppers)

4 medium green, yellow, or red bell peppers
1 cup uncooked brown rice or barley
2 cups vegetable broth or water
2 Tablespoons tomato juice
1 Tablespoon red wine or red vinegar
1/2 cup silken tofu
1/2 cup dried cranberries or raisins
1/4 cup chopped walnuts, almonds, or pine nuts
1 teaspoon black pepper
1 teaspoon ground ginger

Preheat oven to 350 degrees. Cut off pepper tops and remove seeds. Put peppers in a small baking pan (glass is better, but metal will work) with 1 inch of cold water.

In a small pan, mix rice and broth or water. Cover, bring to a boil, reduce heat, and allow mixture to simmer until rice is tender, approximately 40 minutes.

In a small frying pan, heat tomato juice and wine or vinegar together, simmering for 2 minutes. Add tofu and continue to heat, stirring, until liquid is absorbed, approximately 5 minutes.

In a medium-sized bowl, combine cooked rice, cranberries, nuts, pepper, ginger, and tofu. Mix well. Stuff (by firmly pressing filling into peppers) and bake, covered, at 350 degrees for 15 minutes, or until peppers are soft and filling is heated.

Total calories per pepper: 333
Total Fat as % of Daily Value: 12%
Protein: 8 g
Carbohydrates: 59 g
Iron: 2 mg
Exchange: 1 Protein + 4 Starch + 1 Fat

Dietary Fiber: 6 g
Fat: 8 g
Calcium: 42 mg
Sodium: 509 mg

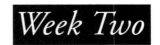

Friday:

Breakfast:
1/4 cup carrot juice
1/2 cup hot whole grain cereal with 1/4 cup peaches
2 rice cakes with 2 Tablespoons peanut butter
8 ounces enriched soymilk

Morning Snack:
1/2 cup sliced pears or apples
3 graham crackers

Lunch:
Vegan hot dog on bun with mustard, catsup,
and pickles or 1/4 cup steamed sauerkraut
1 cup spinach salad with fat-free dressing
8 ounces enriched soymilk

Afternoon Snack:
1/2 cup soy ice cream
topped with 1 teaspoon chopped walnuts or pecans

Dinner:
1 serving **Stuffed Peppers** (page 42)
1/2 cup black beans
Green salad with 1/4 cup sliced, plain beets

Evening Snack:
3 cups air-popped popcorn
sprinkled with 2 teaspoons nutritional yeast
8 ounces enriched soymilk

Freezer Pizza
(Makes 1 serving)

Pizza freezes well, serves as a great place to use leftovers, reheats quickly, and makes a fast breakfast (yes, we all do this sometime!), lunch, dinner, or snack. We've given you a basic recipe; use your imagination (and your leftovers) to enhance it. Pizza crust can be purchased ready-to-use, ready-to-bake, or as a dry mix. You decide which one is most convenient for you. And, of course, you can always use English muffins or bagels instead of crust.

1 six-inch prepared pizza crust
1/2 cup prepared pizza sauce (or canned tomato sauce or salsa mixed with 1 Tablespoon tomato paste)
1/8 cup chopped onions
1/8 cup chopped bell peppers
4 thin slices fresh tomato
1 teaspoon dried basil or 2 teaspoons fresh basil
1 teaspoon dried oregano or 2 teaspoons fresh oregano
2 teaspoons fresh minced garlic or 1 teaspoon granulated garlic

Preheat oven to 400 degrees. Spread sauce evenly on crust. Evenly place onions, peppers, and tomatoes on top of sauce. Sprinkle basil, oregano, and garlic on top of vegetables. Bake pizza for 5 minutes or until vegetables are heated through. Allow to cool thoroughly, then freeze as a whole pizza (a 6-inch pizza is approximately 4 slices) or as individual slices. Remember to label!

Total calories per pizza, using fresh herbs: 859

Total Fat as % of Daily Value: 19%	**Dietary Fiber: 9 g**
Protein: 29 g	**Fat: 12 g**
Carbohydrates: 160 g	**Calcium: 104 mg**
Iron: 10 mg	**Sodium: 2124 mg**

Exchange: 1 Protein + 4 Starch + 2 Vegetable

Vegan Menu for People with Diabetes

Saturday:

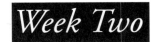

Breakfast:
1/2 cup cranberry-apple juice
1 serving **Corny French Toast** (page 18)
8 ounces enriched soymilk

Morning Snack:
1/2 cup baked sweet potato
topped with 1/4 cup crushed pineapple

Lunch:
1 cup frozen vegan ravioli
with tomato sauce
1/2 cup veggie sticks
1 cup enriched soymilk

Afternoon Snack:
1/2 cup baked sweet potato
with 1/2 cup soft or silken tofu
mixed with 2 teaspoons of maple syrup

Dinner:
1 serving **Freezer Pizza** (page 44)
with 2 ounces vegan pizza pepperoni
1/2 cup mango and grape salad

Evening Snack:
1/2 cup baked winter squash
8 ounces enriched soymilk

Garbs and Carbs
(Makes 2 servings)

1-1/2 cups canned garbanzo beans, drained
1/2 cup chopped celery
1/2 peeled and chopped cucumber
1/4 cup chopped carrots
1/2 cup chopped zucchini or yellow squash
1 chopped green onion
2 Tablespoons chopped fresh parsley
1/8 cup vinegar
2 teaspoons lemon juice
2 teaspoons oil
1/8 teaspoon black pepper

Toss all the ingredients together in a bowl and marinate for at least 1 hour before eating.

Total calories per serving, using zucchini: 247

Total Fat as % of Daily Value: 13%	Dietary Fiber: 12 g
Protein: 9 g	Fat: 8 g
Carbohydrates: 37 g	Calcium: 97 mg
Iron: 4 mg	Sodium: 457 mg

Exchange: 1 Protein + 2 Starch

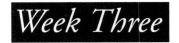

Sunday:

Breakfast:
1 cup melon slices
1 serving (3/4 cup) **Apple Oatmeal** (page 34)
8 ounces enriched soymilk

Morning Snack:
1/2 cup seasonal fresh fruit salad
1/4 cup fat-free granola

Lunch:
1 serving **Garbs and Carbs** (page 46)
1/2 cup steamed broccoli
8 ounces soymilk

Afternoon Snack:
1/2 cup plain soy yogurt with
chopped cucumbers, onions, tomatoes
3 Tablespoons soynuts

Dinner:
1 serving **Oktoberfest Kraut and Beans** (page 49)
2 vegan hot dogs

Evening Snack:
3 cups popcorn
spinkled with 2 Tablespoons nutritional yeast
Fruit Smoothie:
made with 8 ounces enriched soymilk
and 1/2 cup berries

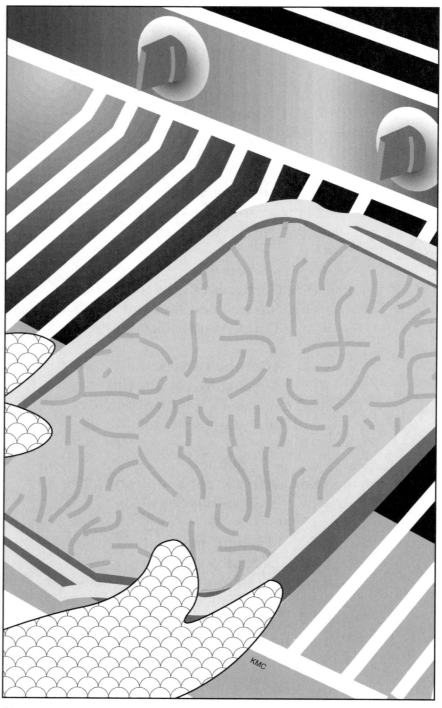

Vegan Menu for People with Diabetes

Oktoberfest Kraut and Beans
(Makes 2 servings)

this recipe is used on page 47

1-1/2 cups canned or fresh sauerkraut
1-1/2 cups canned baked beans
1/4 cup water
2 teaspoons prepared mustard
1 teaspoon caraway seeds

Preheat oven to 400 degrees. Place sauerkraut in strainer or colander. Rinse with cold water and allow sauerkraut to drain.

In a medium-sized baking dish, combine sauerkraut, beans, water, mustard, and caraway seeds. Mix well. Bake for 10-12 minutes or until thoroughly heated.

Total calories per serving: 206
Total Fat as % of Daily Value: 3%
Protein: 10 g
Carbohydrates: 44 g
Iron: 1 mg
Exchange: 1 Protein + 3 Starch

Dietary Fiber: 13 g
Fat: 2 g
Calcium: 141 mg
Sodium: 1465 mg

Lentil-Spinach Pilaf
(Makes 3 servings)

Use canned lentils to speed up preparation.

Vegetable oil spray
2 cups chopped fresh spinach or 1 cup frozen chopped
   spinach, thawed and drained
1 minced garlic clove
3/4 cup cooked lentils (start with 1/3 cup uncooked
   lentils; canned, drained, lentils are fine, too)
1 Tablespoon chopped fresh parsley or 2 teaspoons
   dried parsley
1/4 teaspoon cumin
1/4 teaspoon pepper

Spray a large frying pan with oil and heat. Add spinach
and garlic. Cook, stirring, until spinach is wilted and hot,
approximately 2 minutes. Add lentils, parsley, cumin,
and pepper. Stir until heated through, approximately 3
minutes. Do not overcook, as the spinach will lose its
terrific flavor and texture.

*Note: Cooked soy beans, butter beans (baby limas), and
white beans may be used instead of or in combination
with the lentils.*

Total calories per serving: 72
Total Fat as % of Daily Value: 1%
Protein: 6 g
Carbohydrates: 12 g
Iron: 3 mg
Exchange: 1 Protein + 1 Vegetable

Dietary Fiber: 5 g
Fat: 1 g
Calcium: 52 mg
Sodium: 32 mg

Vegan Menu for People with Diabetes

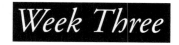

Monday:

Breakfast:
1/2 cup orange/pineapple juice blend
1 bagel spread with 2 Tablespoons nut butter
8 ounces enriched soymilk

Morning Snack:
1 medium banana
2 rice cakes

Lunch:
1 average serving **Tangy Tofu Salad** (page 36)
6 whole wheat crackers
1/2 cup sliced tomato with fresh basil
8 ounces enriched soymilk

Afternoon Snack:
1/2 cup soy ice cream
spinkled with 2 teaspoons nutritional yeast

Dinner:
1 serving **Lentil-Spinach Pilaf** (page 50)
2/3 cup brown rice
1 baked pear

Evening Snack:
1/2 cup baked sweet potato
topped with 2 Tablespoons soy yogurt
8 ounces enriched soymilk

Kitchen Sink Minestrone

(Makes 3 servings)

1-1/2 cups vegetable broth or tomato juice
1/4 cup uncooked pasta
3/4 cup frozen mixed vegetables
1 cup canned chopped tomatoes (with juice)
3/4 cup cooked kidney beans
1 teaspoon granulated garlic
1 teaspoon dried basil or 2 teaspoons fresh basil

Place all the ingredients in a medium-sized saucepan. Bring to a boil. Reduce heat, cover, and simmer until pasta is cooked and vegetables are heated through, approximately 20 minutes.

Note: Try chopping firm tofu and tossing it into the pot during the last 5 minutes of cooking. Use your leftover fresh and frozen vegetables and beans in this soup. If you have leftover cooked pasta, omit the uncooked pasta and add 3/4 cup cooked pasta during the last 10 minutes of cooking.

Total calories per serving, using vegetable broth: 134

Total Fat as % of Daily Value: 2%	Dietary Fiber: 3 g
Protein: 7 g	Fat: 1 g
Carbohydrates: 27 g	Calcium: 122 mg
Iron: 2 mg	Sodium: 564 mg

Exchange for 1-1/2 servings: 1 Protein + 1 Starch + 1 Vegetable + 1 Fruit

Vegan Menu for People with Diabetes

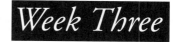

Tuesday:

Breakfast:
1 medium orange, tangerine, or peach
3/4 cup cold whole-grain cereal
1/2 English muffin spread with
1 teaspoon vegan margarine
8 ounces enriched soymilk

Morning Snack:
1/2 cup fat-free veggie chips
1 medium apple

Lunch:
1 cup tofu and 1 cup bell peppers,
sautéed in 2 teaspoons olive oil
1/2 cup sliced carrots
Rice Pudding: made with 1/3 cup cooked rice,
8 ounces enriched soymilk, and sugar-free pudding mix

Afternoon Snack:
1/2 cup soy yogurt with 2 Tablespoons chopped fruit
3 graham crackers

Dinner:
1-1/2 servings **Kitchen Sink Minestrone** (page 52)
with 1/2 cup garbanzo beans

Evening Snack:
3 graham crackers with
2 Tablespoons peanut butter
8 ounces enriched soymilk

One Dish Potato Bar

(Makes 1 serving)

this recipe is used on page 56

This is really a leftover dish. Prepare one or two extra baked potatoes the next time you choose them for dinner.

1 baked potato
1/4 cup cooked beans
2 teaspoons salsa or pizza sauce
1 teaspoon chopped onions
1 teaspoon chopped bell peppers
1 Tablespoon canned or thawed frozen cut corn

Cut baked potato in half, lengthwise. Scoop out potato, being sure to keep the shells intact.

In a small bowl, mix and mash together the beans, salsa or sauce, onions, peppers, and corn. Fill potato shells. Microwave on high for 3 minutes or until hot, or cover and bake at 400 degrees for 7 minutes or until hot.

Total calories per serving, using red kidney beans and salsa: 221

Total Fat as % of Daily Value: 1%	**Dietary Fiber: 9 g**
Protein: 8 g	**Fat: 1 g**
Carbohydrates: 48 g	**Calcium: 19 mg**
Iron: 2 mg	**Sodium: 38 mg**

Exchange: 1 Protein + 3 Starch

Asian Noodle Bowl

(Makes 2 servings)

this recipe is used on page 57

1-1/4 cups cooked noodles, chilled (start with 1/2 cup uncooked noodles)
1/4 cup shredded green cabbage
1/8 cup sliced radishes
3/4 cup diced tofu or wheat gluten
2 teaspoons minced fresh garlic

1 teaspoon minced fresh ginger
1 Tablespoon vegetable oil
1 teaspoon soy sauce
2 Tablespoons cashews or peanuts

In a large serving bowl, toss noodles, cabbage, radishes, tofu or wheat gluten, garlic, and ginger until combined. Add oil and soy sauce. Mix to combine. Garnish with nuts before serving.

Total calories per serving, using tofu and peanuts: 407
Total Fat as % of Daily Value: 31%   Dietary Fiber: 6 g
Protein: 23 g   Fat: 20 g
Carbohydrates: 37 g   Calcium: 180 mg
Iron: 12 mg   Sodium: 187 mg
Exchange: 3 Protein + 1 Fat + 2 Starch + 1 Vegetable

Garlic and Rosemary Sweet Potatoes
(Makes 2 servings)

this recipe is used on page 57

1 large sweet potato (about 1 pound), peeled
  and wedged
1 teaspoon dried rosemary
1 teaspoon granulated garlic
1 Tablespoon melted vegan margarine or oil

Preheat oven to 425 degrees. Toss potato with rosemary and garlic. Arrange potatoes in a single layer on a baking sheet. Drizzle with margarine or oil. Bake for 30 to 40 minutes, turning at least once, until potatoes are tender. Serve warm.

Total calories per serving: 146
Total Fat as % of Daily Value: 9%   Dietary Fiber: 3 g
Protein: 2 g   Fat: 6 g
Carbohydrates: 22 g   Calcium: 30 mg
Iron: 1 mg   Sodium: 78 mg
Exchange: 1 Starch + 1 Fat + 1 Vegetable

Wednesday:

Breakfast:
1/3 cup cranberry juice cocktail
1/2 cup hot whole grain cereal
1 slice toast spread with 1 teaspoon vegan margarine
8 ounces enriched soymilk flavored with
1/2 teaspoon almond extract

Morning Snack:
3/4 cup frozen berries
1/2 cup pretzels

Lunch:
1/2 cup carrot and raisin salad
2 veggie burgers on 1/2 bun with tomato,
lettuce, radish, sprouts, mustard, and/or ketchup
8 ounces enriched soymilk

Afternoon snack:
1/2 cup sugar-free vanilla pudding mixed with
2 Tablespoons chopped dried apricots or cherries

Dinner:
1 serving **One Dish Potato Bar** (page 54)
1/2 cup tofu cubes
1/2 cup spinach salad
1 cup melon cubes

Evening Snack:
1/2 English muffin spread with
2 teaspoons soy cream cheese
8 ounces enriched soymilk

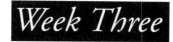

Thursday:

Breakfast:
1/2 cup orange juice
3/4 cup cold whole grain cereal
1 small bran muffin
8 ounces enriched soymilk

Morning Snack:
1/2 cup fat-free pita chips
1/3 cup grape juice

Lunch:
1/2 cup tomato soup
1 serving **Asian Noodle Bowl** (page 54)
8 ounces enriched soymilk

Afternoon Snack:
1/2 cup soy yogurt
sprinkled with 2 teaspoons nutritional yeast

Dinner:
1 serving **Garlic and Rosemary Sweet Potatoes**
(page 55)
with 1 cup baked tofu
1 fresh peach or apricot

Evening Snack:
1 rice cake with 2 Tablespoons peanut butter
8 ounces enriched soymilk

Better Than Beef Stew
(Makes 4 servings)

3/4 cup cubed onions
4 peeled carrots, thickly sliced
1 cup washed and thickly sliced button mushrooms
2 baking potatoes, peeled and cubed
3 minced garlic cloves
1 cup vegetable broth
1/4 cup tomato paste
1/4 cup white wine or 1/4 cup vegetable broth plus
    1 Tablespoon vinegar
1 Tablespoon dried parsley
1 pound tempeh or seitan (flavored is okay), cubed

Preheat oven to 350 degrees. Place all ingredients, except tempeh or seitan, in a medium-sized roasting pan. Cover and allow mixture to bake until all veggies are tender, at least 1 hour. Add tempeh or seitan, recover, and allow dish to stew for an additional 30 minutes.

Total calories per serving, using tempeh: 379
Total Fat as % of Daily Value: 15%   Dietary Fiber: 11 g
Protein: 26 g   Fat: 9 g
Carbohydrates: 52 g   Calcium: 152 mg
Iron: 4 mg   Sodium: 305 mg
Exchange: 3 Protein + 3 Starch + 1 Vegetable

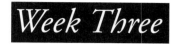

Friday:

Breakfast:
1/2 cup apricot nectar
2 *Breakfast Pizzas:* made with 1-1/2 ounces vegan cheese melted on 2 English muffin halves spread with1 teaspoon vegan margarine
8 ounces enriched soymilk

Morning Snack:
1/2 cup grapes
5 vanilla wafers

Lunch:
1 cup bean chili
1/2 cup cucumber sticks
8 ounces enriched soymilk

Afternoon snack:
1/2 cup fat-free veggie chips

Dinner:
1 serving **Better Than Beef Stew** (page 58)
1/2 banana, sliced and tossed with 1/4 cup orange juice

Evening Snack:
1/2 cup pretzels
8 ounces enriched soymilk

Baked Beans Quesadillas
(Makes 3 whole quesadillas)

If you don't have vegan cheese, a possible substitute would be mashed tofu.

Vegetable oil spray
3 six-inch vegan corn tortillas, cut in half
1 cup canned baked beans*
1 cup shredded vegan cheese
3 Tablespoons chopped fresh cilantro or parsley
For garnish, as desired: chopped fresh tomatoes, chopped or sliced chilies or green bell peppers, additional shredded vegan cheese, and/or sliced black olives

Place 3 tortilla halves on a clean work surface. Spray one side with oil. Turn sprayed side down. Place 1/3 cup beans in the center of three of the tortilla halves. Top beans with vegan cheese and cilantro. Cover with remaining tortilla halves. Spray tops with oil.

Preheat oven to 400 degrees. Spray baking sheet with oil. Place quesadillas on sheet and bake (no need to turn) for 8-10 minutes or until golden. To barbecue the quesadillas instead, grill on each side until golden brown and crisp. To fry them, spray a large frying pan with oil and cook on each side for 3 minutes, or until each side is golden. Serve with garnish, as desired.

*Canned baked beans with barbecue flavor, or add 2 Tablespoons barbecue sauce into the beans to add flavor.

Total calories per quesadilla, using cilantro, but without garnish: 150

Total Fat as % of Daily Value: 3%	**Dietary Fiber: 6 g**
Protein: 7 g	**Fat: 2 g**
Carbohydrates: 30 g	**Calcium: 135 mg**
Iron: 1 mg	**Sodium: 339 mg**

Exchange: 1 Protein + 2 Starch

Vegan Menu for People with Diabetes

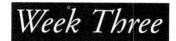

Saturday:

Breakfast:
1/2 broiled red grapefruit
topped with 2 teaspoons maple syrup
2 slices **Corny French Toast** (page 18)
8 ounces enriched soymilk

Morning Snack:
1 medium baked apple
3 ginger snaps

Lunch:
Green salad with fat-free dressing
1 **Baked Beans Quesadilla** (page 60) with salsa
8 ounces enriched soymilk

Afternoon Snack:
Fruit Smoothie: made with 8 ounces enriched soymilk,
2 ounces soft or silken tofu, and 1/2 cup berries
1/4 cup fat-free granola or cold cereal

Dinner:
1 serving **Creamy Carrot Soup** (page 62)
Sandwich: made with 2 ounces fake meat
on 2 slices whole grain bread
spread with 1-1/2 Tablespoons vegan mayonnaise

Evening Snack:
2 breadsticks

Creamy Carrot Soup
(Makes 4 servings)

this recipe is used on page 61

1 pound peeled and thinly sliced carrots
1 cup carrot juice (canned or fresh)
1 teaspoon vegan margarine
2 teaspoons orange juice concentrate
1 teaspoon curry powder
2 cups carrot juice
1 teaspoon lemon zest
1 cup silken tofu

In a large pot, simmer carrots, carrot juice, vegan margarine, concentrate, and curry powder until almost all the liquid has evaporated, approximately 45 minutes.

In a blender or food processor, purée cooked carrots, carrot juice, lemon zest, and tofu and process until very smooth. Refrigerate soup for at least 2 hours or freeze until ready to eat.

Note: Serve this cold soup on a hot night or heat it and serve it hot on a chilly night!

Total calories per serving: 135
Total Fat as % of Daily Value: 5%
Protein: 5 g
Carbohydrates: 23 g
Iron: 1 mg
Dietary Fiber: 4 g
Fat: 3 g
Calcium: 102 mg
Sodium: 146 mg
Exchange: 1/2 Protein + 1 vegetable + 1 Fruit

Revved-Up Oatmeal
(Makes 1 cup)

this recipe is used on page 65

3/4 cup cooked instant oatmeal
1 teaspoon dry sweetener (if desired)
1 Tablespoon raisins
1 Tablespoon wheat germ
1/4 cup soy or rice milk (vanilla-flavored, if you like)

Combine all ingredients in a microwave-safe bowl and heat for 2 minutes on high or until thoroughly heated. Or combine all ingredients in a pot and cook over medium heat, stirring for 5 minutes or until heated.

Total calories per 1 cup serving, using plain soymilk: 240
Total Fat as % of Daily Value: 8%
Protein: 12 g
Carbohydrates: 36 g
Iron: 2 mg
Exchange: 1-1/2 Starch + 1/4 Milk

Dietary Fiber: 5 g
Fat: 4 g
Calcium: 30 mg
Sodium: 20 mg

Apple Yogurt
(Makes 3/4 cup)

this recipe is used on page 65

1/2 cup unflavored or berry-flavored soy yogurt
1 Tablespoon apple butter
1 Tablespoon unsweetened applesauce
1/2 teaspoon ground cinnamon

In a small bowl, combine all the ingredients. Eat right away or store in the refrigerator until ready to eat. Use as a topping for pancakes or instead of milk for cold cereal.

Total calories per 3/4 cup serving: 220
Total Fat as % of Daily Value: 17%
Protein: 10 g
Carbohydrates: 28 g
Iron: 12 mg
Exchange: 1/2 Protein + 1/2 Starch + 1 Fat

Dietary Fiber: 3 g
Fat: 11 g
Calcium: 200 mg
Sodium: 19 mg

Green and Creamy Soup
(Makes 4 servings)

Vegetable oil spray
1/2 cup chopped onion
1/4 cup celery
3 cups vegetable broth
1/4 cup dried split peas, rinsed
1 bay leaf
1 cup diced zucchini or yellow squash (thawed, frozen squash will work)
1/2 teaspoon dried basil
1 cup thawed, frozen chopped spinach, drained
1 Tablespoon chopped fresh parsley

Heat a medium-sized saucepan and spray with oil. Sauté onions and celery until soft, approximately 2 minutes. Add vegetable broth, split peas, and bay leaf. Bring to a quick boil, reduce heat, and cover. Simmer for 30 minutes. Add squash and basil and simmer for 5 minutes.

Remove bay leaf and place soup in a blender. Blend until smooth. Put soup back in pot, add spinach and parsley, and heat for 5 minutes. Serve soup hot or allow it to cool before freezing.

Total calories per serving: 84
Total Fat as % of Daily Value: 2%
Protein: 6 g
Carbohydrates: 15 g
Iron: 2 mg

Dietary Fiber: 4 g
Fat: 2 g
Calcium: 67 mg
Sodium: 793 mg
Exchange for 1-1/2 servings: 1 protein + 1 Starch

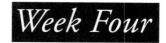

Sunday:

Breakfast:
1 medium baked apple
1 cup **Revved-Up Oatmeal** (page 63)
4 ounces enriched soymilk

Morning Snack:
3/4 cup **Apple Yogurt** (page 63)

Lunch:
1-1/2 servings **Green and Creamy Soup** (page 64)
1/2 cup pasta with tomato sauce
1 cup carrot sticks
8 ounces enriched soymilk

Afternoon Snack:
Parfait: made with 1/2 cup silken tofu,
2 Tablespoons chopped nuts
and 1 Tablespoon maple syrup

Dinner:
1 cup vegetable broth with 1/3 cup cooked rice
1 serving **Put Together In Ten Minutes Casserole**
(page 66)
1 slice watermelon

Evening Snack:
1/2 cup pita chips with
1-1/2 ounces melted vegan cheese
8 ounces enriched soymilk

Put Together in Ten Minutes Casserole

this recipe is used on page 65

(Makes 2 servings)

You can probably prepare this casserole in even less time!

1/2 cup chopped celery
1/4 cup chopped onions
1 Tablespoon soy sauce
1 teaspoon granulated garlic
1/2 teaspoon ground ginger
3/4 cup diced firm tofu, tempeh, or seitan
10-ounce can vegan mushroom soup
1/3 cup frozen peas
1/2 cup vegan chow mein noodles (the crunchy ones)

Preheat oven to 350 degrees. In a baking dish, combine all ingredients except chow mein noodles. Mix until combined. Top with noodles and bake for approximately 45 minutes or until lightly browned and bubbly.

Note: Dare we tell you that if no chow mein noodles are to be found, you can use smashed potato or corn chips?

Total calories per serving: 293
Total Fat as % of Daily Value: 22%   **Dietary Fiber: 6 g**
Protein: 20 g   **Fat: 15 g**
Carbohydrates: 25 g   **Calcium: 218 mg**
Iron: 12 mg   **Sodium: 1187 mg**
Exchange: 3 Protein + 1 Starch + 1 Vegetable

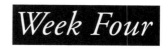

Monday:

Breakfast:
1/2 cup orange juice
1/2 cup cold cereal
1/2 bagel spread with 1 teaspoon vegan margarine
8 ounces enriched soymilk

Morning Snack:
1/2 cup baked sweet potato
topped with 1/4 cup crushed pineapple

Lunch:
Mixed Bean Burrito: made with 1 tortilla
filled with salsa mixed with 1/2 cup beans
1 cup coleslaw with vegan mayonnaise
8 ounces enriched soymilk

Afternoon Snack:
1/2 cup chocolate sugar-free pudding
with 1/2 cup berries
3 Tablespoons soy nuts

Dinner:
2 veggie hot dogs or burgers
Grilled portobello mushroom over 2/3 cup brown rice
1/2 cup steamed carrots
1/2 cup pineapple and 1/4 cup cherries

Evening Snack:
5 vanilla wafers
with 2 teaspoons soy cream cheese
8 ounces enriched soymilk

Zucchini, Green Bean, and Potato Stew
(Makes 2 servings)

Vegetable oil spray
1/4 cup chopped onions
1 cup cut green beans (fresh or thawed frozen)
1/4 teaspoon red pepper flakes
1/2 cup sliced zucchini (fresh or thawed frozen)
1 cup baking potato, peeled and cubed
1/4 cup chopped fresh parsley
1-1/2 cups chopped canned tomatoes, not drained
 (or use one 8-ounce can)

Heat a large frying pan and spray with oil. Add onions and sauté until soft, approximately 2 minutes. Add green beans and pepper flakes and continue to sauté until onions are translucent, approximately 3 minutes. Add zucchini, potato, and parsley, and toss to mix. Add tomatoes. Bring to a fast boil, lower heat, cover, and simmer, stirring frequently, until potatoes are tender, approximately 40 minutes.

Total calories per serving: 129
Total Fat as % of Daily Value: 2%
Protein: 5 g
Carbohydrates: 28 g
Iron: 2 mg
Exchange: 2 Starch

Dietary Fiber: 6 g
Fat: 1 g
Calcium: 97 mg
Sodium: 279 mg

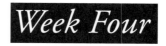

Tuesday:

Breakfast:
1/2 cup apricot nectar
1/2 cup hot whole grain cereal
2 rice cakes spread with 1 teaspoon vegan margarine
8 ounces enriched soymilk

Morning Snack:
1/2 cup cinnamon applesauce
3 ginger snaps

Lunch:
1 average serving **Tangy Tofu Salad** (page 36)
3 saltines
1/2 cup carrot and raisin salad
8 ounces enriched soymilk

Afternoon Snack:
1/2 cup soy yogurt
topped with 2 Tablespoons granola
and 3 Tablespoons soy nuts

Dinner:
1 serving **Zucchini, Green Bean,
and Potato Stew** (page 68)
2 ounces vegan sausage
1 sliced pear

Evening Snack:
3 graham crackers
8 ounces enriched soymilk

Raisins and Brown Rice
(Makes 3 servings)

Enjoy this kind of sweet, kind of savory dish.

1-1/2 cups water
1/2 cup uncooked brown rice
1/4 cup raisins
1/4 cup slivered or chopped almonds
2 teaspoons onion powder
1 teaspoon dried parsley
1/8 teaspoon cinnamon
1 teaspoon vegan margarine

In a medium-sized saucepan, bring water to a boil. Add rice, raisins, almonds, onions, parsley, and cinnamon. Reduce heat, cover, and cook for approximately 45 minutes or until liquid is absorbed. Stir in margarine and serve hot.

Total calories per serving: 220
Total Fat as % of Daily Value: 10%
Protein: 5 g
Carbohydrates: 37 g
Iron: 1 mg
Exchange: 2-1/2 Starch + 1 Fat

Dietary Fiber: 3 g
Fat: 6 g
Calcium: 44 mg
Sodium: 20 mg

Vegan Menu for People with Diabetes

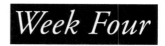
Wednesday:

Breakfast:
1/2 banana in 1/4 cup orange juice
1/2 cup oatmeal
1/2 bagel with 1 teaspoon vegan margarine
8 ounces enriched soymilk

Morning Snack:
1/2 cup peach nectar
3 cups popcorn
sprinkled with 2 teaspoons nutritional yeast

Lunch:
2 veggie burgers with shredded carrots,
sliced cucumbers, and chopped cabbage
1/4 cup veggie chips
8 ounces enriched soymilk

Afternoon Snack:
1/2 cup soy ice cream with 1/2 cup berries

Dinner:
1 cup baked tofu or Tofurky™
1 serving **Raisins and Brown Rice** (page 70)
1/2 cup swiss chard
1/4 cup fruit salad

Evening Snack:
4 whole wheat crackers
8 ounces enriched soymilk

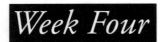

Thursday:

Breakfast:
1/2 cup pink grapefruit sections
2 *Breakfast Pizzas:* 2 English muffin halves,
1-1/2 ounces vegan cheese, 1 teaspoon vegan margarine
8 ounces enriched soymilk

Morning Snack:
1/2 cup pretzels
1/3 cup grapes

Lunch:
Pita with 2 ounces fake meat,
sliced tomato, diced onion, bell peppers or
chili peppers, and 1-1/2 Tablespoons vegan mayonnaise
8 ounces enriched soymilk

Afternoon Snack:
1/2 cup baked veggie chips
with 2 teaspoons soy cream cheese

Dinner:
2 servings **Baked Pasta and Peppers** (page 30)
Baked apple

Evening Snack:
2 breadsticks
with 1/2 cup hummus

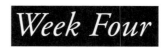

Friday:

Breakfast:
1/2 cup fresh or frozen mango or papaya
1/2 cup hot cereal
1 rice cake with 1 teaspoon vegan margarine
8 ounces enriched soymilk

Morning Snack:
1/2 banana
1 small bran muffin

Lunch:
1 cup vegan ravioli with tomato sauce
1/2 cup Romaine lettuce
with 2 Tablespoons croutons
8 ounces enriched soymilk

Afternoon Snack:
1/2 cup baked sweet potato
with 1/2 cup tofu
and 2 teaspoons maple syrup

Dinner:
3/4 serving **Quick Cajun Rice and Beans** (page 74)
with 1/4 cup soy crumbles
1/2 cup steamed cauliflower

Evening Snack:
3 cups air-popped popcorn
3 Tablespoons soy nuts
8 ounces enriched soymilk

Quick Cajun Rice and Beans
(Makes 2 servings)

this recipe is used on page 73

Vegetable oil spray
1/2 cup chopped onions
1/2 cup chopped green bell pepper
1 minced garlic clove
1/2 cup (4 ounces) soy sausage or soy crumbles
1 cup canned chopped tomatoes
1 cup vegetable broth
1 cup instant rice (such as Minute Rice)
1/2 teaspoon black pepper
1/2 teaspoon thyme
1/2 teaspoon oregano
1 cup canned white beans (such as great Northern or butter beans), drained
1 cup canned red beans, (such as kidney beans), drained
Tabasco or hot sauce, as desired

Heat a large pot and spray with oil. Add onion, bell pepper, and garlic and sauté until soft, approximately 2 minutes. Add soy sausage or crumbles and cook for 1 minute. Add tomatoes, broth, and rice. Bring to a fast boil, reduce heat to simmer, and add black pepper, thyme, and oregano. Cover pot and cook for 4 minutes. Stir in beans and continue to cook until beans are hot and all liquid is absorbed. Add Tabasco™ and serve.

Total calories per serving: 475
Total Fat as % of Daily Value: 7%	**Dietary Fiber: 21 g**
Protein: 25 g	**Fat: 4 g**
Carbohydrates: 87 g	**Calcium: 156 mg**
Iron: 7 mg	**Sodium: 750 mg**

Exchange for 3/4 serving: 2 Protein + 4 Starch

Vegan Menu for People with Diabetes

Breakfast Potato Burritos
(Makes 3 burritos)

this recipe is used on page 77

Vegetable oil spray
1 cup frozen hash browns, thawed
1/2 cup cooked soy crumbles* See glossary.
1/4 cup chopped bell pepper
1/4 cup chopped green onions
1 chopped chili (if desired)
4 Tablespoons firm tofu, crumbled
3 ten-inch flour tortillas

Spray a large frying pan with oil. Brown potatoes. Add crumbles, pepper, onions, and chili and sauté until vegetables are soft, approximately 3 minutes. Add tofu and cook, tossing until well combined and heated through. Divide mixture into thirds and fill tortillas.

Note: Sliced mushrooms can be used instead of soy crumbles. These burritos can be assembled the night before and then heated in a 350 degree oven for 10 minutes the next day. The burritos can also be frozen.

Total calories per burrito 412
Total Fat as % of Daily Value: 23%   **Dietary Fiber: 5 g**
Protein: 13 g   **Fat: 15 g**
Carbohydrates: 59 g   **Calcium: 147 mg**
Iron: 6 mg   **Sodium: 482 mg**
Exchange: 1 Protein + 4 Starch + 2 Fat

Hot Apples and Sweet Potatoes
(Makes 4 servings)

What a way to get your fruit in the morning! This makes a great hot breakfast and could also be a sweet side dish for spicy meals.

1/2 cup vegan dry sweetener
1/2 teaspoon nutmeg
1/2 teaspoon cinnamon
1/2 teaspoon ground ginger
3/4 cup raw sweet potatoes, peeled and sliced thinly
1/8 cup canned crushed pineapple, drained
3/4 cup green apples, peeled, cored, and sliced very thinly
1/2 cup granola
1/8 cup raisins, dried cranberries, or dried cherries
Vegetable oil spray

Preheat oven to 375 degrees. In a small bowl, mix sweetener, nutmeg, cinnamon, and ginger. In a medium-sized bowl, combine remaining ingredients except for oil spray. Combine spice and apple mixtures and mix well.

Spray a baking sheet with oil. Spread apple/sweet potato mixture on baking sheet and cover with foil. Bake for 45 minutes or until potatoes and apples are soft. Eat while warm.

Total calories per serving, using raisins: 223
Total Fat as % of Daily Value: 4%	**Dietary Fiber: 3 g**
Protein: 2 g	**Fat: 3 g**
Carbohydrates: 50 g	**Calcium: 26 mg**
Iron: 1 mg	**Sodium: 28 mg**

Exchange per 1/2 serving: 1 Starch + 1 Fruit

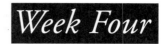

Saturday:

Breakfast:
1 **Breakfast Potato Burrito** (page 75)
1/2 cup seasonal fruit salad
8 ounces enriched soymilk

Morning Snack:
1/2 serving **Hot Apples and Sweet Potatoes** (page 76)

Lunch:
3/4 serving **Tofu Scramble** (page 34)
1/2 cup braised spinach
1 steamed tortilla
8 ounces enriched soymilk

Afternoon Snack:
1/2 cup soy ice cream

Dinner:
1 serving **Pasta in Paradise** (page 38)
1 fresh tangerine, peach, or apricot

Evening Snack:
1/2 baked potato with salsa
and a sprinkle of nutritional yeast
8 ounces enriched soymilk

Glossary

Chocolate Pudding: See "Pudding."

Fake Meat or Deli Slices: Also known as meat substitutes, fake meat or deli slices can be found in the refrigerator and freezer case of your local food market. Numerous items fall into this food category including veggie burgers and hot dogs, mock chicken and turkey, ground round (a substitute for chopped meat), mock steak, veggie sausage, etc. Many of these products are made from soy or wheat gluten combined with other ingredients.

Nutritional Yeast: Nutritional yeast sometimes is fortified with vitamin B12. Red Star company prodouces a "Vegetarian Support Formula" nutritional yeast that contains vitamin B12. This is a good source of B12 for vegans. Read the labels. Not all nutritional yeasts contain vitamin B12, and some are not vegan (they may contain whey). You can sprinkle nutritional yeast on hot or cold cereal, on soups, in baking batters and doughs, on cooked vegetables, and in casseroles.

Pudding: Sugar-free pudding comes as a dry mix, both instant and non-instant, which is then prepared with regular or lowfat soy, rice, or grain milk. Very few of these mixes contain milk solids, whey, or other dairy products. Generally, they consist of a combination of artificial sweetener, corn starch (that's what makes the thickness), and artificial flavors and color. Available brands vary from region to region. Some brands are Sweet 'n Low, Estee, and Hains.

Smoked Seitan: Look for flavored seitan in the refrigerated section of your natural foods market. You can also use barbecue-flavored seitan if you can't find smoked.

Soy Crumbles: Usually found in the refrigerator case of natural foods stores and some supermarkets, soy crumbles can be used to make tacos, sloppy Joe sandwiches, etc.

Soy Sour Cream: Non-dairy vegan sour cream can be found in natural foods stores, Kosher supermarkets, and some other markets. One popular brand is Tofutti™.

Vanilla Pudding: See "Pudding."

TVP (Textured Vegetable Protein): TVP is made from soy flour that is compressed until the protein fibers change in structure. It comes dried and it is rehydrated in hot water. TVP is available in different sizes, so if you wanted to make a stew-like dish, you could use the larger chunks, compared to the smaller chunks, which would be good for chili and sloppy Joes. TVP is available in most natural food stores and may come in bulk, which is cheaper.

Vegan: A vegan does not eat any animal products including meat, fish, poultry, eggs, dairy products, honey, etc. A vegetarian does not eat meat, fish, or poultry.

Vegan Dry Sweetener: Some cane sugar is processed through bone char filters. See <www.vrg.org/jouornal/vj97mar/973sugar.htm> for more information.

Vegan Graham Crackers: These are graham crackers that do not contain honey or any dairy products. You can find them in some supermarkets.

Guide to Substitutions

Once you've become familiar with the exchanges, you will be able to replace suggested menu items with menu items more to your liking. The list starting on the next page is a breakdown of exchanges for recipes included in this book, as well as snacks, meat substitutes, and other food items.

Substituting for your taste preferences is easy. If you aren't crazy about tomatoes, then Wonder Gazpacho won't be your favorite. One serving of Wonder Gazpacho is equal to one fruit exchange, so instead of having gazpacho, choose 1/2 cup orange juice, or 17 grapes, or 3/4 cup fresh strawberries. As we said before, please try not to make many substitutions within the menus, as the days have been set up to incorporate a great deal of nutritional variety, and subsitutions undermine those considerations.

Recipes:

(Exchanges are per serving unless otherwise noted. Page number refers to where recipe appears in the meal plan.)

3/4 cup Apple Oatmeal (2 Starch + 2 Fat); page 33 and 47

3/4 cup Apple Yogurt (1/2 Protein + 1 Starch + 1 Fat); page 65

Asian Noodle Bowl (3 Protein + 1 Fat + 2 Starch + 1 Vegetable); page 57

1 Baked Beans Quesadilla (1 Protein + 2 Starch); page 61

2 servings Baked Pasta and Peppers (2 Protein + 1 Vegetable + 2 Starch + 2 Fat); page 31 and 72

Better than Beef Stew (3 Protein + 3 Starch + 1 Vegetable); page 59

1 Breakfast Potato Burrito (1 Protein + 4 Starch + 2 Fat); page 77

1 Cinnamon, Apple, and Raisin Pancake (3 Starch + 1 Fruit + 1 Fat); page 29

Corn and Potato Chowder (2 Protein + 1 Vegetable + 2 Starch); page 27

1 slice Corny French Toast (1-1/2 Starch + 1/2 Fat); page 45

2 slices Corny French Toast (3 Starch + 1 Fat); page 19

Creamy Carrot Soup (1/2 Protein + 1 Vegetable + 1 Fruit); page 61

Freezer Pizza (1 Protein + 4 Starch + 2 Vegetable); page 44

Garbs and Carbs (1 Protein + 2 Starch); page 47

Garlic and Rosemary Sweet Potatoes (1 Starch + 1 Fat + 1 Vegetable); page 57

1-1/2 servings Green and Creamy Soup (1 Protein + 1 Starch); page 65

1/2 serving Hot Apples and Sweet Potatoes (1 Starch + 1 Fruit); page 77

1-1/2 servings Kitchen Sink Minestrone (1 protein + 1 Starch + 1 Vegetable + 1 Fruit); page 53

1 cup Lentil Chili (2 Starch + 1 Vegetable + 1 Very Lean Protein); page 19

Lentil-Spinach Pilaf (1 Protein + 1 Vegetable); page 51

Oktoberfest Kraut & Beans (1 Protein + 3 Starch); page 47

One Dish Potato Bar (1 Protein + 3 Starch); page 56

Pasta In Paradise (1 Protein + 1 Fat + 4 Starch); page 39 and 77

Power Chili (1 Starch + 2 Protein); page 37

Put Together In Ten Minutes Casserole (3 Protein + 1 Starch + 1 Vegetable); page 65

3/4 serving Quick Cajun Rice and Beans (2 Protein + 4 Starch); page 73

Raisins and Brown Rice (2-1/2 Starch + 1 Fat); page 71

1 cup Revved-Up Oatmeal (2 Starch + 1/2 Milk); page 65

1-1/2 servings Salsa Black Bean Salad (2 Protein + 1 Vegetable + 1/2 Fruit + 2 Starch); page 39

Stuffed Peppers (1 Protein + 4 Starch + 1 Fat); page 43

1 average serving Tangy Tofu Salad (1 Protein + 1/2 Vegetable + 1/2 Fat); page 51 and 69

1 hearty serving Tangy Tofu Salad (2 Protein + 1 Vegetable + 1 Fat); page 37

3/4 serving Tofu Scramble (4 Protein + 1 Starch); page 77

Tofu Scramble (5 Protein + 1 Starch); page 33

Wonder Gazpacho (1 Fruit); page 33

Zucchini, Green Bean, and Potato Stew (2 Starch); page 69

Snacks:

1-1/2 Tablespoons soy nuts (1/2 High-Fat Protein + 1/2 Starch)

1-1/2 Tablespoons vegan mayonnaise (1 Fat)

1/2 cup soy ice cream (1 starch + 2 Fat)

1 cup vegetable bean soup (1 Protein + 1 Starch + 1 Vegetable)

2 teaspoons vegan soy cream cheese (1 Fat)

1-1/2 ounces vegan cheese (1 Starch + 1 Fat)

2 slices vegan pizza (2 Starch + 2 Protein + 1 Vegetable)

6 ounces soy yogurt (1 Starch + 1/2 Fruit)

Meat Substitutes:

6 strips vegan soy bacon (2 Lean Protein)

2 veggie burgers (2 Lean Protein + 1 starch)

1 veggie hot dog (1 Lean Protein)

1 ounce vegan deli slices (1 Lean Protein)

1/4 cup prepared TVP (1 Lean Protein)

2 ounces smoked seitan (1 Lean Protein + 1 Starch)

2 ounces vegan fake meat (2 Lean Protein)

Miscellaneous Substitutes:

8 ounces enriched soymilk = 1 ADA milk exchange (120 calories)

1/2 cup fresh, frozen, or canned fruit = 1 ADA fruit exchange (60 calories)

2 Tablespoons dried fruit = 1 ADA fruit exchange (60 calories)

1 slice of bread equivalent, such as 1/2 bagel, 1/2 hamburger bun, 3 cups low- or non-fat popped popcorn, or 1 tortilla = 1 ADA starch exchange (80 calories)

1/3 cup cooked rice or 1/2 cup cooked pasta = 1 starch exchange

2 plain (without spread) breadsticks, 3/4 ounces pretzels, 3 gingersnaps, or 3 graham cracker squares = 1 ADA starch exchange

1/2 cup cooked or 1 cup raw vegetables = 1 ADA vegetable exchange

1/2 cup cooked beans, 1/3 cup tofu, or 2 Tablespoons nut butters = 1 very lean protein exchange + 1 starch exchange

Guide to Resources
from The Vegetarian Resource Group

The following resources can be purchased from The Vegetarian Resource Group, PO Box 1463, Baltimore, MD 21203. You can order online at <www.vrg.org>, or charge your order over the phone by calling (410) 366-8343 between 9 am and 5 pm EST Monday through Friday.

Shipping and Handling Charges:

Orders under $25	$6 ($10 for Canada/Mexico)
Orders over $25	Free in continental U.S.
Foreign orders	Inquire first

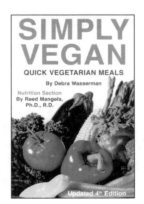

Simply Vegan
Quick Vegetarian Meals

The immensely popular *Simply Vegan*, by Debra Wasserman and Reed Mangels, PhD, RD, is much more than a cookbook. It is a guide to a non-violent, environmentally sound, humane lifestyle. It features over 160 vegan recipes that can be prepared quickly, as well as an extensive nutrition section. The chapters cover topics on protein, fat, calcium, iron, vitamin B12, pregnancy and the vegan diet, and raising vegan kids. Additionally, the book includes sample menus and meal plans. There is also information on cruelty-free shopping by mail, including where to buy vegan food, clothing, cosmetics, household products, and books.

Available for $15. (224 pages)

Meatless Meals
for Working People

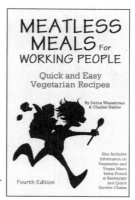

Meatless Meals For Working People, by Debra Wasserman and Charles Stahler contains over 100 delicious fast and easy recipes, plus ideas which teach you to be a vegetarian within your hectic schedule using common convenient vegetarian foods. This handy guide also contains a spice chart, party ideas, information on quick service restaurant chains, and much more.

Available for $12. (192 pages)

Vegan Meals for
One or Two

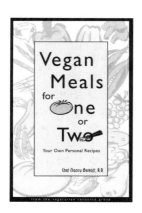

Each recipe in *Vegan Meals for One or Two*, by Nancy Berkoff, EdD, RD, is designed so that you can realistically use ingredients the way they come packaged from the store when cooking for one or two. Meal planning and shopping information is included, as well as breakfast ideas, one-pot wonders, recipes that can be frozen for later use, grab-and-go suggestions, everyday and special occasion entrées, plus desserts and snacks. Sample recipes include Breakfast Potato Burritos, Lentil-Spinach Pilaf, Almost Thai Spicy Peanut Pasta, Asian Sautéed Eggplant, Quick Tofu Stroganoff, Grilled Sweet Onions, and Baked Pears in Apple Cider Syrup. A glossary is provided.

Available for $15. (216 pages)

Conveniently Vegan
Turn Packaged Foods into Delicious Vegetarian Dishes

CONVENIENTLY
VEGAN
Turn Packaged Foods into
Delicious Vegetarian Dishes

By Debra Wasserman

In *Conveniently Vegan*, by Debra Wasserman, you will learn how to prepare meals with all the new natural foods products in stores today. Features 150 healthy recipes using convenience foods along with fresh fruits and vegetables. Explore creative ideas for old favorites, including Potato Salad, Stuffed Peppers, Quick Sloppy Joes, "Hot Dogs" and Beans, Lasagna, Chili, Bread Pudding, and Chocolate Pie. Menu ideas, food definitions, and product sources.

Available for $15. (208 pages)

Vegan Microwave Cookbook

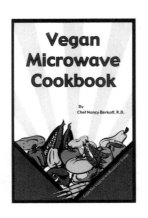

Vegan Microwave Cookbook

By
Chef Nancy Berkoff, R.D.

Vegan Microwave Cookbook, by Nancy Berkoff, RD, offers over 165 recipes that can be prepared in a microwave oven. Many of the recipes will take under 10 minutes to cook. Others may be more appropriate for entertaining. Helpful advice includes: Converting Traditional Recipes to the Microwave, Microwave Baking and Desserts, Breakfast in a Snap, Curries and Casseroles, and Suggestions for Holidays and Parties. Sample dishes include Cilantro-Marinated Tofu, Basic "Meat" Balls, Microwave Lasagna, Pizza Potatoes, Coriander Kale with Slivered Carrots, Corn and Chili Muffins, and much more.

Available for $16.95. (288 pages)

ORDER USING THE FORM ON PAGE 92

Vegan Handbook

Vegan Handbook contains over 200 vegan recipes, including the basics, international cuisine, and gourmet dishes. Also features information on sports nutrition, a seniors' guide to good nutrition, feeding vegan kids, menus, guide to leather alternatives, vegetarian history, and much more. This is an 8-1/2 x 11-inch book!

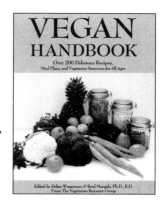

Available for $20. (256 pages)

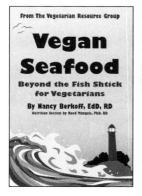

Vegan Seafood
Beyond the Fish Shtick for Vegetarians

According to a national Vegetarian Resource Group Poll conducted by Harris Interactive, almost 15% of Americans say they never eat fish or seafood. For all of you, and others who would like alternatives to fish, Chef Nancy Berkoff has created unique and good-tasting dishes including Mango Salad with Avocado and "Shrimp," "Crab" Enchiladas, "Tuna" Noodle Casserole, Ethiopian-Style "Shrimp" and Sweet Potato Stew, and Spicy "Fish" Cakes. After using this book, you'll agree with millions of vegetarians and say: SEA ANIMALS — DON'T EAT THEM!

Available for $12. (96 pages)

OR ONLINE AT < WWW.VRG.ORG/CATALOG >

The Lowfat Jewish Vegetarian Cookbook

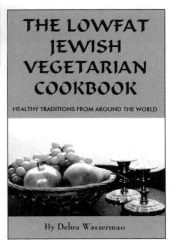
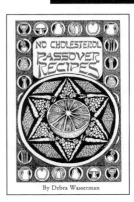

Vegan Passover Recipes

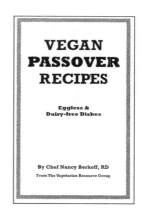

Vegan Passover Recipes, by Nancy Berkoff, RD, RD, offers many eggless and dairy-free options for a healthy and great-tasting Festival of Freedom, including soups, salads, side dishes, sauces, entrées, and desserts. All recipes are suitable for Ashkenazi Eastern European Jewish tradition, which does not use beans or rice. Sample dishes include French Onion Soup, Pear and Apple Slaw, Minted Carrots with Chilies, Apricot and Tomato Sauce, Coconut Curry Over Greens, Spinach and Okra Stew, Moroccan Roasted Eggplant and Pepper Salad, Strawberry Sorbet, Cinnamon Matzah Balls, Pizza Casserole, Vegetarian Kishka, and much more.

Available for $6. (48 pages)

Vegetarian Journal's Guide to Food Ingredients

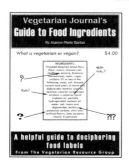

This guide is very helpful in deciphering ingredient labels. It lists the uses, sources, and definitions of hundreds of common food ingredients. The guide also states whether the ingredient is vegan, typically vegan, vegetarian, typically vegetarian, non-vegetarian, or typically non-vegetarian.

Available for $6. (28 pages)

OR ONLINE AT < WWW.VRG.ORG/CATALOG >

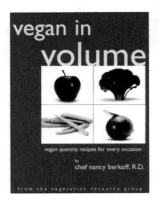

Vegan in Volume
Vegan Quantity Recipes for Every Occasion

Vegan in Volume, by Nancy Berkoff, RD, is a 272-page book. It has 125 quantity recipes for every occasion. Chef Nancy Berkoff offers help with catered events, weddings, birthdays, college food service, hospital meals, restaurants, dinner parties, etc. She shares her knowledge of vegan nutrition, vegan ingredients, menus for seniors, breakfast buffets, desserts, cooking for kids, and much more.

Available for $20. (272 pages)

Vegetarian Journal's Guide to Leather Alternatives

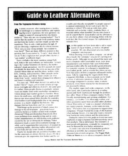

Besides not eating animals, you may not want to wear them! This guide is very helpful in locating non-leather items including shoes, belts, and bags. You'll even find sources for cruelty-free computer cases, Ipod and cell phone holders, skate boarding shoes, and much more. This comprehensive list includes store locations and online mail-order resources.

Available for $5. (8 pages)

ORDER USING THE FORM ON PAGE 92

Vegan Menu for People with Diabetes

Subscribe to Vegetarian Journal

The practical magazine for those interested in health, ecology, and ethics.

<u>Inside each issue find</u>:

Nutrition Hotline—answers to your questions about vegetarian diets.

Lowfat Vegan Recipes—quick and easy dishes, international cuisine, and gourmet meals.

Natural Food Product Reviews

Scientific Updates—recent scientific papers relating to vegetarianism.

Vegetarian Action—individuals and groups incorporating vegetarianism into their lives and communities.

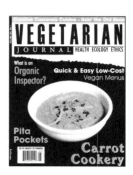

VEGETARIAN JOURNAL (ISSN 0885-7636) is published quarterly by the independent Vegetarian Resource Group.

Yes! I want to receive *Vegetarian Journal!*

Name: _____

Address: _____

City: _____ State: _____ Zip:_____

☐ Payment Enclosed (check or money order)

☐ Please charge my (circle one) MasterCard / Visa:

  # _____ Expires: ____ /____

In the U.S., send $20 for one year of the quarterly *Vegetarian Journal*; in Canada and Mexico, please send $32; other foreign subscribers, please send $42 in U.S. funds or via MasterCard or Visa. Send payment and subscription information to The Vegetarian Resource Group, PO Box 1463, Baltimore, MD 21203. Or fax this form to (410) 366-8804. You can order online at <www.vrg.org/journal/subscribe.htm>. Please e-mail vrg@vrg.org with any questions.

OR ONLINE AT < WWW.VRG.ORG/CATALOG>

Order More Copies of Vegan Menu for People with Diabetes for $10 each!

Use or photocopy the form below to order *Vegan Menu for People with Diabetes* or any other books or publications featured in this book.

Vegetarian Resource Group *Order Form*

Name: _____

Address: _____

City: _____ State: _____ Zip: _____

Phone: _____ E-mail: _____

Item:	Quantity:	Price:	Subtotal:
_____	_____	$_____	$_____
_____	_____	$_____	$_____
_____	_____	$_____	$_____
_____	_____	$_____	$_____

Subtotal: $_____

SHIPPING INFORMATION
For orders under $25, add $6 in the U.S. and $10 in Canada and Mexico. Shipping is free for orders over $25 in the continental U.S. For all other foreign orders, please inquire first.

Shipping: $_____

MD Residents Add 5% Sales Tax: $_____

Donation: $_____

Total: $_____

☐ Payment Enclosed (check or money order)

☐ Please charge my (circle one) MasterCard / Visa:

\# _____ Expires: ____ / ____

Send order information and payment to The Vegetarian Resource Group, PO Box 1463, Baltimore, MD 21203. Or fax this form to (410) 366-8804. You can order via telephone at (410) 366-8343 Monday through Friday from 9 am to 5 pm EST or online at <www.vrg.org>. Please e-mail vrg@vrg.org with any questions.

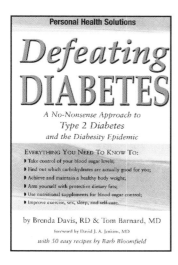

Brenda Davis, RD, and Tom Barnard, MD, authors of *Defeating Diabetes,* have written a book that clearly explains how a plant-based diet focusing on simple, whole foods can be a most effective tool for defeating diabetes. The book includes a thoroughly researched section on the relationship between diabetes and diet, ideas for weight control, a food guide, and a 7-day menu plan. There are also 50 vegan recipes.

Available for $14.95. (280 pages)

The Whole Foods Diabetic Cookbook, by Patricia Stevenson and Michael Cook with information on diabetes and nutrition by Patricia Bertron, RD, features close to 90 vegan recipes for breakfast, breads, salads, sandwiches, soups, main dishes, vegetables, and even desserts. Recipes use common foods and are generally simple to prepare.

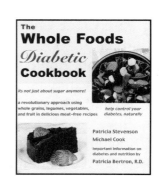

Information on diabetic exchanges for each recipe is included, as well as an overview of diabetes, a discussion of the health benefits of a vegetarian diet, and suggestions for meeting nutrient needs.

Available for $14.95. (160 pages)

ORDER USING THE FORM ON PAGE 92

Index

Vegan Menu for People with Diabetes

Join The Vegetarian Resource Group and Support our Work!

The Vegetarian Resource Group (VRG) is a non-profit organization dedicated to educating the public on vegetarianism and the interrelated issues of health, nutrition, ecology, ethics, and world hunger.

Our health professionals, activists, and educators work with businesses and individuals to bring about healthy changes in your school, workplace, and community. Registered dietitians and physicians aid in the development of nutrition-related publications and answer member or media questions about the vegetarian diet. The Vegetarian Resource Group sponsors an annual college scholarship for graduating high school seniors. Two awards of $5,000 each are given (see <www.vrg.org>).

To join The Vegetarian Resource Group and receive *Vegetarian Journal* send $20 to VRG, PO Box 1463, Baltimore, MD 21203 or call (410) 366-8343; 9 am to 5 pm EST Monday-Friday.

To Order More Copies of Vegan Menu for People with Diabetes

Send $10.00 for each book to VRG, PO Box 1463, Baltimore, MD 21203 or call (410) 366-8343; 9 am to 5 pm Monday-Friday.

Visit our Website <www.vrg.org>

Find vegan recipes, travel tips, the latest updates on vegetarian nutrition, and much more with just a click of your mouse! Sign up for VRG-News, our online newsletter, or join our parent's list where vegetarian families share ideas.

This book is printed on recycled paper!